A Good
Fat

BOOK YOUR PLACE ON OUR WEBSITE AND MAKE THE READING CONNECTION!

We've created a customized website just for our very special readers, where you can get the inside scoop on everything that's going on with Zebra, Pinnacle and Kensington books.

When you come online, you'll have the exciting opportunity to:

- View covers of upcoming books

- Read sample chapters

- Learn about our future publishing schedule (listed by publication month *and author*)

- Find out when your favorite authors will be visiting a city near you

- Search for and order backlist books from our online catalog

- Check out author bios and background information

- Send e-mail to your favorite authors

- Meet the Kensington staff online

- Join us in weekly chats with authors, readers and other guests

- Get writing guidelines

- AND MUCH MORE!

Visit our website at
http://www.kensingtonbooks.com

DHA

A Good Fat
Essential for Life

JAMES J. GORMLEY

Kensington Books
Kensington Publishing Corp.
http://www.kensingtonbooks.com

This publication and product is designed to provide accurate and authoritative information with regard to the subject matter covered. The purchase of this publication does not create a doctor-patient relationship between the purchaser and the author, nor should the information contained in this book be considered specific medical advice with respect to a specific patient and/or a specific condition. In the event the purchaser desires to obtain specific medical advice or other information concerning a specific person, condition, or situation, the services of a competent professional should be sought.

The author and publisher specifically disclaim any liability, loss, or risk, personal or otherwise, that is or may be incurred as a consequence, directly or indirectly, of the use and application of any of the information contained in this book.

KENSINGTON BOOKS are published by

Kensington Publishing Corp.
850 Third Avenue
New York, NY 10022

First Printing: July, 1999
10 9 8 7 6 5 4 3 2 1

Printed in the United States of America

To my wife, Juana, and our children,
Natalia and Julian—
my deepest love, always.

ACKNOWLEDGMENTS

Just as DHA is *essential for life*, my family is essential to everything in my life.

I want to thank my parents—Edward Patrick Gormley and Audrey Mary Keller-Gormley—for having always believed in me. Little do they know how deeply I've always believed in them.

I want to thank my wife, Juana, for having put up with me for all these years! Her infectious dynamism and determination have inspired me.

My deepest thanks to my children—Natalia Marie and Julian Edward—for gracing Juana and me with their unbounded imagination and irrespressible love.

A note of thanks to Lee Heiman, of Kensington Publishing, who said "Yes, let's do it!" before I had even finished proposing the DHA book idea to him.

Appreciation is also due to Angela Tsetsis, David Kyle, Ph.D., Gregg Lampf, and Claire Mullins, at Martek, each of whom were kind enough to help me locate studies and researchers; they even were nice enough to let me use illustrations for this book. I applaud Martek, and its CEO, Henry Linsert, Jr., for having the courage—and tenacity—to believe in a natural fat that may help our world prevent "nutritional Armageddon."

Contents

Foreword
By Leo Galland, M.D., Director,
Foundation for Integrated Medicine,
author, *Power Healing*

The discovery of the essential fatty acids (EFAs) and their role in human health was one of the most important scientific discoveries of the twentieth century. Extensive research has shown that disturbances in the dietary intake of EFAs, or in their metabolism within the body, play an important role in the development of most of the chronic diseases that plague our society.

The most significant problem is a marked decline in our consumption of the *omega–3* EFAs which are found in green vegetables, oily fish, flax, soy, walnuts, and wild game. This widespread omega–3 deficiency is aggravated by the increasing use of processed vegetable oils and by suboptimal consumption of those vitamins, minerals, and antioxidants which the body depends upon for properly utilizing EFAs.

EFA imbalance has two major consequences. The body uses EFAs to build the membranes of all cells. A lack of omega–3 EFAs produces cell membranes that are stiff and do not function properly. EFAs are also used by the body to make a group of super-hormones called prostaglandins (PGs) and leukotrienes (LTs). An imbalanced intake of EFAs can distort the production of PGs and LTs in the body, causing dysfunction or disease.

Restoring the right nutritional balance of EFAs for each person is one of the cardinal goals of nutritional medicine. It has been a major focus in my medical practice for the past twenty years.

In this well-referenced and readable book, James Gormley makes an important contribution to public understanding of EFA balance. After clearly explaining the nature of essential fats and their roles in the body, he focuses on one particular EFA—docosahexaenoic acid, or DHA—which was long neglected in nutritional studies.

DHA is the longest and most complex of the EFAs and is especially concentrated in the brain. Ordinarily, if you consume enough of the omega–3 EFAs from food, your body will automatically produce all the DHA it needs. Most Americans, however, do not consume an adequate supply of omega–3 foods and many lack some of the nutrients needed for proper EFA metabolism. For some of these people, supplementation of the diet with DHA may be the only means to preserving and restoring health.

Gormley describes the sources of DHA and its use as a nutritional supplement, citing important scientific publications as he does so. He describes the many disorders in which DHA supplementation may be beneficial, but this book is not only about DHA. It provides a perspective on the impact that EFAs, in general, have on health and points toward the not-so-distant future in which the specific EFA needs of individuals will be assessed scientifically, so that individually targeted essential fatty acid therapy will be possible for everyone.

Introduction

April 3, 1997, was a red letter day for brain and total body health. It was on this day a press conference was held at New York Hospital-Cornell Medical Center. It was called "Keeping Your Brain In Shape: New Insights Into DHA."

Even more specifically, it was a monumental day for nutrition. Some of the world's leading experts spoke about the research on this humble, little omega–3 fat with the big name: docosahexaenoic acid—DHA, for short.

Frankly, I was floored by what I saw and heard. Along with several research papers, slides of children with fat-metabolism "defects" were shown, slides that made me cry. Then they were followed by slides of these same children after undergoing dietary supplementation with DHA. There were astonishing improvements!

I became so taken with DHA and the research done on it that I wrote my June 1997 editorial (in *Better Nutrition* magazine) on DHA itself. I titled the piece "DHA and the Excitement of New Research."

My excitement about DHA research hasn't subsided. Nor has the ever-growing interest in DHA among scientists, researchers, consumers, baby formula makers, and supplement manufacturers subsided—it has only increased!

Fortunately, at this point, the research supporting the use of DHA is, by now, incontrovertible. The "DHA Locomotive" cannot be slowed, halted, or moved off course.

The Federal Drug Administration (FDA), which has still to approve the substance, will now have no other choice but to allow formula makers to include DHA and arachidonic acid in all baby formula products sold to U.S. consumers.

In the meantime, we can arm ourselves with the treasure trove of research linking DHA supplementation to neurological development, brain health, retinal function, and protection from a variety of diseases and disorders. And that is what I hope to help you do by way of this book.

Overall, though, this book is meant as a message of *balance*. A balance of fats in our diet is what's critical. Overloading on any one component—including DHA—to the detriment or exclusion of others is definitively *not* what I will suggest.

Again, I wish to point us toward a balance of all fats in the diet, a balance which existed, by and large, prior to the cholesterol crazes and low-fat/fat-free mania of the middle portion of this century which is now, and thankfully so, drawing to a close.

In the new millennium, I hope that we will see a food supply free from genetically engineered products, irradiation, toxic pesticides, and nutritional imbalance. Although reducing our toxic burden is critical, so is having an American diet balanced in all major food components, including fats.

If this book will only help bring a consciousness of fat balance into the larger equation of rational nutrition, then it will have fulfilled its mission.

Because, truly, DHA is: *essential for life.*

James Gormley
Riverdale, New York
November 1998

PART I

▼

Fats in Context

Looks as if we're becoming a nation of Jack Sprats. Why? Mainly, because mass-market food producers know that it's cheaper to make foods with virtually no fat, or at least foods with virtually no critical omega–3 fatty acids, foods missing a fat that's essential for life: docosahexaenoic acid (DHA).

We also know that the right balance of fats in our prenatal and postnatal diets helps to determine the health of our brain and retina.

We will now journey on an overview of the various diseases related to faulty processing of, and/or dietary deficiencies of, DHA. And as we do so, we'll take a glimpse at the research into DHA, which we'll look at more completely in Parts II through V, including:

1. Diseases of the mind (depression, schizophrenia, and Alzheimer's disease)
2. Attention deficit hyperactivity disorder (ADHD)
3. Dyslexia and retinitis pigmentosa
4. Metabolic and peroxisomal disorders (LCHADD, Zellweger syndrome, and more)
5. Diseases of immunity, inflammation, and allergy
6. Cardiovascular disease
7. Maternal, prenatal, and infant nutrition

In fact, we will see how close as a nation we have come to the brink of "Nutritional Armageddon."

Fortunately, we will also see that science is on the

verge of comprehending a "new paradigm in nutrition," one which recognizes the wisdom of:

- Balancing the fats in our diets
- Eliminating poor quality (tropical oils) and semi-toxic alternatives (partially hydrogenated oils, including margarine)
- Increasing our consumption of microalgae-source DHA and other omega–3 fats

....

CHAPTER 1

Polyunsaturated fatty acids: fats in context

> Jack Sprat could eat no fat,
> His wife could eat no lean;
> And so betwixt them both,
> They licked the platter clean

Poly-un *what?* That's what I said when I first came across the term. To fully understand the term we'll start with the fat part, and work back to the beginning. Quite simply, fats are one of six groups of nutrients that are essential for life. The other five groups are: protein, carbohydrates, vitamins, minerals, and water.

Before we get into polyunsaturated fats and their relations, however, let's recall a few of the critical and essential benefits of dietary fats.

What's the Big, Fat Deal?

Fats are energy generators

Fats, which are made up of many kinds of fatty acids, are involved in an incredible array of body activities. Their most immediate function is to hold on to energy until it's needed. Fats also provide the main flavor and texture of foods and allow our bodies to absorb vitamins A, D, and E.

Fats hold everything together

Each and every cell is covered by a membrane that performs a variety of functions essential for life: cell membranes keep the cellular contents intact, maintain each cell's shape and flexibility, and control the passage of things in—and out of—each cell.

At this point, it's important to know that the way each membrane is built is powerfully influenced by fatty acids. In some membranes—like those in the skin and those which form protective sheaths around nerves—specific fatty acids provide a water barrier and an insulating layer.

Fats are key components of body processes

Certain fatty acids—such as those in cell membranes—are *absolutely essential* for the production of chemical messengers that start up, or keep on top of, many things which go on in the body, including: cell growth and division, blood pressure and blood coagulation (platelet stickiness), immune reactions, and tissue inflammation.

But What's a Fatty Acid?

I answered that question this way in a 1997 talk I gave in Kingston, New York, at the Hudson Valley Health, Fitness & Nutrition Expo:

The technical answer involves carbon chains, organic acid groups, and hydrogen atoms. But, mostly, fatty acids are oils that make up our foods, make up structures in our bodies and cells, and are necessary for life.

In fact, fatty acids are the foundation of all fats and oils, whatever the source—in food or our body. Fats, called "lipids" by scientists, are solid at room temperature; oils are lipids that are liquid at the same temperature. Fats and oils are composed of building blocks called "fatty acids."

Now if you look at a fatty acid molecule, this is what you will find: the "fatty" end of the molecule is water-insoluble (or "hydrophobic": water-avoiding) and oil-soluble ("lipophilic," or water-loving), meaning that this end does not dissolve in water and is most happy in fatty regions of our bodies—the membranes and tissues. This fatty section, or chain, is mostly made up of carbon and hydrogen atoms, ending in what is called a methyl (–CH) group.

The other end of the molecule is its "acid" part. And the acid part, or end, of the molecule is, as we might expect, a water-soluble (or "hydrophilic": dissolving in water) organic acid called a carboxyl (–COOH) group, which does not dissolve in oil—remember though that it does dissolve in water.

Back on the chain gang?

Fatty acids are like chains. They're different, one from another, in the length of the chain, and in the number and position of fixed, or "rigid," links (the "carbon position" of the first double bond). When all the links are flexible, the fatty acid is called "saturated." Fatty acids with one rigid link are dubbed "monounsaturated"; fats with more than one of these links are called "polyunsaturated."

Monounsaturated fatty acids (MUFAs) and polyunsaturated fatty acids (PUFAs)

PUFAs can be further broken down into special "families," according to the position of the first rigid link. With each family different from all others, the three most important for health have the link at the third, sixth, and ninth position: omega–3 fats (including DHA-rich land and sea sources—flax and fish oil), omega–6 fats (including most seed oils), and omega–9 fats.

Fatty acids all have different quantities of carbon atoms in their "fatty chain," but most of the fatty acids range between four carbons (such as the butyric acid in butter) and 24 carbons (found in some fish oils and brain tissue). Scientists number the carbon atoms in fatty acid chains using the omega numbering system, starting with an omega–1—at the beginning of the methyl end—and ending with an omega–18—at the border of the carboxyl end.

The long and short of it

According to this mumbo-jumbo sytem, DHA is written like this: 22:6n3. Although this looks a little too much like math, what this means is that DHA is a long-chain (more than 14 carbons in its chain), 22-carbon-long polyunsaturated fatty acid with six (6) double-bonds. It's called an omega–3 because the first double-bond occurs at the third (3) carbon from the omega end.

A "short-chain" fatty acid is a saturated fat with six, or fewer, carbon atoms in its chain—an example is butyric acid, a four-carbon fat found in butter. A "medium-chain" fatty acid has six to 12 carbon atoms—two examples are caprylic acid (with eight) and capric acid (with 10).

Virtually all of what we'll be looking at in this book will be: omega–3 *long-chain* polyunsaturated fats, DHA specifically.

"The name's bond"

Hydrogen and carbon atoms in fatty acids play house by sharing electrons with each other. Each pair of shared electrons forms what is called a "single bond," one which marries a carbon with a carbon. All of the fatty acids we'll be talking about are of the polyunsaturated variety, meaning, in part, that they have two, or more, double-bonds (more to come on this later).

Saturated Fats

The carbons of fatty acids linked by single bonds are "saturated." Each of the carbon atoms establishes four bonds with other carbons and holds as many hydrogen atoms as it physically can—making it "saturated with hydrogen," or just *saturated*. Most of these fats are solid, or semisolid, at room temperature.

Animal fats "pump up the volume" when it comes to saturated fats. Although most of us don't think it, some vegetables and nuts are pretty high in saturated fats as well (coconut, palm, avocado, peanut, and walnut). On the other hand, these foods have recently been criticized for their fat profiles. But as with diet and with individual foods, it's the whole "fat picture" that matters most. In this sense, then, the truth about almonds, for example, is somewhat different from what you might think. Almonds are only made up of 5–9% saturated fat. The rest of their profile looks like this: 65% monounsaturated omega–9 [oleic acid] and 26% polyunsaturated omega–6 [linoleic acid].

Saturated fat sources at-a-glance:

- butter
- animal fat
- coconut oil
- palm oil
- palm kernel oil
- cocoa butter

Unsaturated and Monounsaturated Fats

In organisms (animals and plants), "unsaturated" fats are produced from saturated fats after our bodies insert one, or more, double bonds into these fats and take out two hydrogen atoms. These unsaturated fatty acids are both less stable and more active (chemically) than saturated fatty acids, which usually just sit there.

A mono*unsaturated fat*—which has one carbon-to-carbon (C=C) double-bond—tends to be fluid and to not stick together.

Examples of monounsaturated oils are:

- olive (82% monounsaturated omega–9, 8% polyunsaturated omega–6 [linoleic acid], and 10% saturated fat)
- canola/grapeseed (60% monounsaturated omega–9, 24% polyunsaturated omega–6, 10% polyunsaturated omega–3 [alpha-linolenic], and 6% saturated fat.
- Although rather high in saturated fat, peanut and avocado are classed as monounsaturated oils.

Two "new" oils out on the market also fit in the monounsaturated category: "high-oleic" safflower and "high-oleic" sunflower oils.

Monounsaturated foods at-a-glance:

- canola oil
- olive oil
- avocado oil
- high-oleic safflower
- high-oleic sunflower

Polyunsaturated Fats

Unsaturated fatty acids with two, or more, double bonds are known as "polyunsaturated," which includes both omega–3 fatty acids (mostly found in ocean-dwelling algae, North Atlantic fish, and dark green vegetables), and omega–6 fatty acids (mostly found in nuts and seed oils).

Polyunsaturated oils are liquid at room temperature and refrigerated. Examples are: flaxseed, corn, soy, sesame, sunflower and safflower oils.

Omega–3 polyunsaturated foods at-a-glance:

- microalgae
- fish oil
- flaxseed oil
- canola/grapeseed oil

Omega–6 polyunsaturated foods at-a-glance:

- safflower oil
- corn oil
- sunflower seed oil
- cottonseed oil
- peanut oil
- sesame oil
- grapeseed oil
- borage oil
- evening primrose

The Brink of Nutritional Armageddon?

Cis to trans—*from nice to nasty in one easy step*

Very suspiciously coinciding with the anti-fat craze of the 1960s and 1970s (from which we still haven't completely recovered), food manufacturers had a problem.

Chart 1.1
The Primary Essential Fatty Acid Groups
& Dietary Sources

Group	Parent fatty acid	(PU)/FA	Sources
POLYUNSATURATED GROUP			
Omega–3	Alpha-linolenic		Green plants, ocean-dwelling microalgae, plankton, soybeans, *esp. flaxseed, candlenut, hemp & pumpkin seed*
	Alpha-linolenic	EPA (eicosapen-taenoic)	Marine oils, fish, *esp. Chinese water snake oil*
	Alpha-linolenic	DHA (docosa-hexaenoic)	Ocean-dwelling microalgae
Omega–6	Linoleic acid		Nuts, seeds, vegetable & seed oils, *esp. safflower & sunflower*
	Linoleic acid	AA (arachidonic)	Meats
	Linoleic acid	GLA (gamma-linolenic)	Borage, black currant seed, evening primrose
		DGLA (dihomogamma-linolenic)	Mother's milk
MONOUNSATURATED GROUP			
Omega–7		POA (palmitoleic)	Tropical oils, *esp. coconut & palm kernel oils*

Chart 1.1 (cont.)

Group	Parent fatty acid (PU)/FA	Sources
Omega–9	OA (oleic)	Land-animal fats & butter, and plant/nut oils, *esp. olive, almond, peanut, pecan, cashew, filbert & macadamia*

SATURATED GROUP & SOURCES:

- **Stearic acid:** Mutton, beef, butter, pork, shea nut butter, cocoa butter and chocolate
- **Palmitic acid:** Tropical fats from coconut, palm and palm kernel
- **Butyric acid:** Butter
- **Arachidic acid:** Peanuts

The mass-market food manufacturers' problem

How to provide more wholesome, clean, and nutritious food for all Americans? No. How to maximize profits by placing the United States on the brink of "nutritional Armageddon"? Yes.

More specifically, their problem was with a primary oil used in the preparation of mass market foods. Corn oil (after losing its natural antioxidants and protective compounds through "refining") then became vulnerable to "oxidation"—spoilage and rancidity—by processing, transportation, and storage. In addition, one of food producers' "desirable food qualities" for oils—firmness—wasn't possible with normal, unadulterated oil.

Their main goals were sixfold:

1. Bring products to the market that have obscenely long shelf-lives.

2. Maximize profits and minimize the costs of ingredients.
3. Reduce spoilage and rancidity.
4. Promote the inclusion of omega–6 seed oils as a supposed benefit for consumers.
5. Use an oil which would give consumers a creamy consistency and flavor, have a firm texture, and be capable of withstanding the massive nutrient-killing heat which faster processing calls for.
6. Maximize profits and minimize the costs of ingredients.

Yes, I know, we already listed number 6 in number 2—that was intentional!

A Soylent Green *solution for our food producers?*

In a certain way, there is a relationship between the two. *Soylent Green* was a 1973 MGM film about twenty-first century society (New York City, in this case) going to extreme measures to feed the masses and reduce overpopulation. In this Richard Fleischer-directed classic, the lead protagonist, Charlton Heston, is horrified when he discovers at the film's conclusion, the "secret ingredient" in the soybean-lentil superfood called "soylent green"—people!

Now, I'm not saying that our masters of manufacturing have resorted to pushing cannibalism to accomplish their goals, but I am saying that they came up with a way to achieve their goals. And their solution, which we'll presently examine, is plenty horrific all on its own.

Hydrogenation—"something wicked this way comes"

Our princes of production discovered that if vegetable oils could be heated, exposed to semitoxic and toxic metals (such as nickel and aluminum), and exposed to hydrogen gas, foods could then achieve almost infinite shelf-life.

In the process, however, the molecular configuration of the hydrogenated fatty acids was (and is) perverted from the natural *cis* position (in which the hydrogen atoms are all on one side of the double bond) to a *trans* position, essentially turning the *cis* molecules into what are called "*trans* fatty acids," plastic fats whose hydrogen atoms are situated on opposing sides of the fat chain.

According to C.K. Chow, in the very revealing book *Fatty Acids in Foods and Their Health Implications,* by about 1980 Americans were consuming an estimated 10 billion pounds of fats and oil a year, of which 60 percent was partially hydrogenated oil—now the most popular *trans* fat around.

The "trans fat" nightmare

In point of fact, trans-fatty acids think that they're saturated fats, unfortunately, and truly act the part. They lower your "good" cholesterol (HDL), increase your "bad" cholesterol (LDL), and reduce the oil's naturally occurring levels of the essential fatty acids—the fats we really need!

Through the process of hydrogenation, the adding of hydrogen to the oil's double-bonds, gives a higher melting point to this "new" trans-fatty acid, achieving the food producers' marketing dream of developing a cheap oil that has both a creamy consistency and a firm texture, not to mention longer shelf life.

Where are these trans fats found? Trans fats are found in mass-market (non-health-food store) varieties of practically everything!: all processed and refined foods, shortening, prepared mixes, deep-fat fried foods, commercial baked goods (including cakes, bread, and cookies), crackers, canned soups and foods, processed cheese, cereals, candies, mass-market oils, snack foods, and, you guessed it, margarine.

In fact, partially hydrogenated oils have about 15–25 percent trans-fatty acids; shortenings have about 26–51 percent. These plastic fats permeate the entire U.S. diet. Nutrition researcher Mary Enig, of the University of Maryland, has analyzed the trans-fat content in more than 600 foods—from puddings and crackers to imitation cheese and chicken nuggets. She concluded that the average American consumes upward of 28 grams of trans fats a day, since these fats easily represent 20 percent of the typical diet. A male athlete consuming 4100 calories a day, for example, could take in nearly 60 grams of trans fats!

Some trans fatty acids, but certainly not of the majority used in processed foods, are produced in the rumen (or stomach) of ruminating animals by microorganisms, and are found "naturally" in certain animal fats, such as beef, and dairy products (butter and cheese).

The 5 percent solution? Not quite, more like the 5 percent *limit*. Studies show that consistently consuming more than 5 percent of our calories in the form of trans fats leads to serious health problems.

Again according to M.G. Enig, in a 1993 edition of *Nutrition Quarterly*, trans-fats and partially hydrogenated oils have been associated with conditions and diseases we can and must avoid in our search for better health, greater vitality, and longevity, including: low infant birth weight, low production and quality of breast milk in women, obesity, abnormal sperm production and lowered testosterone in men, suppression of the immune system, heart disease, heightened levels of harmful cholesterol, prostate disease, and essential fatty acid deficiency.

Research on trans fats. Now the most recent research on trans fats was carried out at the United States Department of Agriculture, Agricultural Research Service

(USDA/ARS), Human Nutrition Research Center, in Beltsville, Maryland.

In this federally funded study, researchers showed that trans fats boosted serum cholesterol just like saturated fat. How tragically ironic. Our masters of manufacturing's "cholesterol friendly" grand solution—those very same trans fats—is just as bad as the saturated fat it is supposed to replace; worse, if we consider the toxic partial-hydrogenation process.

Trans fats cause disease. In another revealing study done in 1993, Walter C. Willett, M.D., Ph.D., chairman of the nutrition department at Harvard University's School of Public Health, found that "positive associations between intake of trans fatty acids and coronary heart disease (CHD) have been observed" in epidemiological data. In fact, Willett has recently said that, of all oils and edible fats, trans fats have the strongest association with the risk of heart disease itself.

Trans fats cause 30,000 deaths each year. Using the backdrop of his own research, and that of Mensink and Katan (1990) and Aro, et al. (1995), Willett wrote on the effects of these perverted fats on cholesterol levels, and the relation of these lipid components to the risk for coronary heart disease: "It can be conservatively estimated that approximately 30,000 deaths per year in the U.S. are attributable to *trans* fatty acids from partially hydrogenated vegetable oil."

If we accept that trans fats should make up no more than 5 percent of total dietary fat intake, then we're in for a rude awakening. L. Litin and F. Sacks evince this most clearly for us in their 1996 *New England Journal of Medicine* article. For in that article, they state that we can reach the "5 percent max" by eating only one doughnut for breakfast, a small order of french fries with lunch, a teaspoon of margarine with dinner, and two cookies for dessert. As Ray Bradbury so perfectly put it: "something wicked this way comes."

Some manufacturers are trying a different way: un-margarines? In all fairness though, some companies have responded to the problem, but only in *their* way. Rather than produce foods with the kind of fats that the body really needs, they have refined the foods they previously marketed and that the body doesn't need, and then repackaged them. I'm speaking here of spreads—whether with expeller-expressed canola oil or stanol esters—that are said to contain *no* trans fats. This isn't bad, of course. Spreads without trans fats does give them the advantage over margarine, but not over the "good fats" (which we'll discuss later in this chapter).

What About Those Polyunsaturated Fatty Acids (PUFAs) Again?

The body can make specific fatty acids from carbohydrates, such as starch and sugar. Two PUFA "parents," however—linoleic acid (omega–6) and alpha-linolenic acid (omega–3)—cannot for all intents and purposes, be produced *in* the body and, like essential vitamins, must be obtained from food and supplements.

These polyunsaturated fatty acids (Chart 1.1) are called essential fatty acids, or EFAs. From these two parent compounds, also necessary for life and health, other essential fatty acids are made.

From "the mother of all omega–6 fats"—linoleic acid—as a starting point, the body can then synthesize the primary members of the omega–6 family: gamma-linolenic acid (GLA), dihomogamma-linolenic acid (DGLA), and arachidonic acid (AA).

From "the mother of all omega–3 fats"—alpha-linolenic acid—the body can then produce these omega–3 PUFAs, for example: eicosapentaenoic acid (EPA), docosahexaenoic acid (DHA), and docosapentaenoic acid (DPA).

What Happens When We Break Down These Fats?

Eicosanoids—The Good, the Bad, and the Inflammatory

Okay, now we know where the fats come from—their ancestry, if you will. But what happens to them as they're broken down by our systems? Good question.

While the answer partly lies in extremely powerful hormone-like compounds, called **eicosanoids**, and members of their family, including **interleukins** (special "glyco"proteins), **prostaglandins** (derived from "good" and "bad" fats), and **leukotrienes** (derived from white blood cells), the story is one of inflammation. Inflammation of what? Our joint tissues, our respiratory system, our vessels, etc.

Now fats play a part here since they break down into "good" and "bad" prostaglandins and influence thereby how these other immune/inflammation players behave: the eicosanoids, interleukins, and leukotrienes as mentioned above.

Is inflammation always bad?

Absolutely not. Inflammation is not always bad and is critical in such areas as wound healing. Inflammation does cause problems, however, when it runs out of control, such as in asthma and severe allergic reaction. In our effort to reduce forms of inflammation that do run out of control, our goal is homeostasis—a state in which a system functions properly and in balance. And this goes even for each and every cell related to inflammation that serves specific, important purposes, depending on need.

Again, problems arise, and diseases can get their start, when we are *not* in a state of homeostasis—when the inflammatory cascade veers out of control, as mentioned—or when inflammation:

1. continues beyond the borders of a specific need (e.g., wound healing);
2. is triggered by natural or toxic environmental causes (e.g., pollen or DDT); or,
3. is pervasive and running rampant, bespeaking a bodily system which is drowning in a reactive sea of synthetic food ingredients, environmental toxins, and internal mediators (like prostaglandins), themselves awash in products and symptoms of an immune system that is redlining at the same time that it has run out of fuel.

Enter Polyunsaturated Fatty Acids

When scientists and physicians think of inflammation, they probably have pro-inflammatory chemicals in mind, such as interluekin–1, leukotriene B4, and prostaglandins. Fats are involved in producing and controlling some of these chemicals. For instance, omega–6 seed oils break down into prostaglandin E1 ("good") and prostaglandin E2 ("bad"). Omega–3 fats, on the other hand, only break down into a "good" prostaglandin, E3. So, in this light, let's turn to a more in-depth discussion of inflammation and immune function via PUFAs.

Inflammation and immune function

Today we know that a diet, or supplementation program, rich enough in omega–3 fatty acids can rein in an immune system that has gone bonkers. Another way omega–3 fats put things back on track is by cutting down on how many leukocytes (white blood cells) are called into action.

Omega–3 fats can prevent inflammation in other ways, too. They can throw a monkey wrench into the production of those pro-inflammatory chemicals produced by cells, **interleukin–1** (IL–1), **leukotriene B4** (LTB4), and a specific series of **prostaglandins**. It looks something like this.

IL-1

Omega–3 fats keep excessive production of IL–1 in check, which is important since an imbalance, or excess, of IL–1 has been tied to a wide array of diseases, including: AIDS, allergies, Alzheimer's disease, asthma, atherosclerosis, chronic obstructive pulmonary disease (COPD), Crohn's disease, multiple sclerosis (MS), psoriasis, rheumatoid arthritis, type–I diabetes, and ulcerative colitis.

LTB4

Omega–3 fats also hold back the body's production of LTB4, which is good since this compound has been specifically linked to such conditions as: asthma, dermatitis, emphysema and bronchitis, inflammatory bowel disease (IBD), psoriasis, rheumatoid arthritis, and ulcerative colitis.

The story of prostaglandins is a little bigger, but we'll just glance at them, as far as they relate to fatty acids in our diet.

Prostaglandins (PGs)

As mentioned, these are physiologically active, hormone-like characters that are found in a whole bunch of different tissues. The skeletal frame of prostaglandins is composed of prostanoic acid, a 20-carbon acid. Again, prostaglandins come in three families, or series: series 1, series 2, and series 3. Series 1 ("good") and series 2 ("bad") come from the omega–6 family of fats, which includes linoleic acid; series 3 prostaglandins ("good"), on the other hand, come from the omega–3 group of fats, which includes eicosapentaenoic acid (EPA).

The "good guys"? Series 1 prostaglandins do a lot of good things for our body. They:

- keep platelets from sticking together excessively (helpful in preventing atherosclerosis);
- remove sodium and excess fluid from the body (via our kidneys);
- relax blood vessels;
- improve circulation;
- lower blood pressure;
- relieve angina;
- help insulin work better (important in diabetes);
- improve nerve function;
- modulate calcium metabolism;
- improve our immune functioning (and that of T cells), and more.

Series 3 prostaglandins made from EPA, prevent arachidonic acid (AA) from being released by cell membranes. In this way, if PGE3s are hanging around, PGE2s decide to keep a really low profile.

PGE2s—Visigoths at the Gates? Series 2 prostaglandins have been criticized of late, with some of that criticism pretty well deserved. In fairness though, we want these wild card PGE2s to be around, especially when we prick a finger with a rusty nail, for example. The swelling, and consequent expansion of blood vessels, allows white blood cells to corner and overcome the inevitable bacterial invasion brought on by these same chemicals.

On the other hand, as the Romans discovered, while one of the Visigoth "barbarians" (like series 2 prostaglandins) you hired to guard your borders may keep *those* entry points pretty safe, the fact that the other 20,000 you hired are now fanning throughout your kingdom pillaging, looting, and otherwise marauding is not bringing a smile to your face. PGE2s are our bodies' own "Visigoths at the Gates."

The "Good Seed" (Oils)

On land, seed begets life. All seeds are "good" in this sense (despite what your weed-pulling gardener told you!). It is, in fact, awe inspiring to consider how much energy, nutrition, and power is poised inside one little seed. Nutrient packed by necessity, the fat content in different seeds and nuts varies considerably—from a low of 4 percent in corn, for example, to a high of nearly 72 percent in macadamia nuts. Nevertheless, of more interest than the total fat content in nuts and seeds is the **fatty acid profile**, what the breakdown, or balance, of different fats looks like for each.

So omega–6 oils are okay, then?

True enough, at least in terms of their fatty acid profile. Aside though, from the fact that the "typical" U.S. diet is completely overbalanced in the ratio of omega–6 fats to omega–3 fats, there are a number of excellent, highly nutritious oils with high levels of omega–6 fats:

- **evening primrose** (81% omega–6, 17% total fat)
- **safflower** (75% omega–6, 59.5% total fat)
- **sunflower seeds** (65% omega–6, 47.3% total fat)
- **hemp** (60% omega–6, 35% total fat)
- **corn** (59% omega–6, 4% total fat)
- **pumpkin seeds** (42–57% omega–6, 46.7% total fat)

Black currant seed and **borage seed** are no slouches, either. In fact, like evening primrose and hemp, borage and black currant are rich in linoleic acid and gamma-linolenic acid (said to be helpful in arthritis and pre-menstrual syndrome [PMS]).

Which Land-Based Oils Are the Best?

Finding which land-based oils are best is somewhat difficult, since "best" depends on what you're looking for. **High quality** and a **balanced fatty-acid profile** though are a couple of important parameters.

Quality. Clearly, we're talking about oils that are un-refined, expeller (mechanically) pressed, and pressed without solvents. They should be freshly processed, quickly (and well) bottled, and speedily delivered to your favorite health food store.

Balanced fatty-acid profile. If we look at those land-based oils (not derived from the sea) which have a balance of different types of fat, then these oils truly stand out:

- **hemp (20% omega–3, 60% omega–6, 12% omega–9)**
- **flax (58% omega–3, 14% omega–6, 19% omega–9)**
- **pumpkin seed (0–15% omega–3, 42–57% omega–6, 34% omega–9)**
- **chia (30% omega–3, 40% omega–6, 12% omega–9)**
- **candlenut/kukui (29% omega–3, 40% omega–6)**

Although the last two, unfortunately, are pretty diffi-cult to obtain, **hemp** is not. With its 3:1 ratio of omega–6 fats to omega–3 fats (and its content of GLA), it's a good land-based oil useful for helping to avoid essential fatty acid deficiency.

We've been talking a lot about oil from land-based sources. Let's take a look at oil from the sea.

Of Fish Oil and Snake Oil

Fish Oil

So I'll just eat a lot of fish and get all the omega–3 fats I'll ever need—right? Not necessarily. Let's take a look at the big picture. Although it is true that Arctic/ North Atlantic fish are very rich in EPA and DHA, it's important to look at EPA-rich fish oil, its negatives and positives—and some alternatives.

The negatives

Brings on vitamin E deficiency. Since fish oil is more vulnerable to oxidation—to turning rancid—than most other fats, the body mobilizes vitamin E to help check oxidizing chain reactions before they get out of control, which then depletes vitamin E stores.

Infants and small children

Although we'll look in greater depth at the omega–3 needs of prenatal infants (as they develop), along with the needs of babies and the needs of children, papers presented at a meeting of the American Oil Chemists' Society, in 1992, reinforce the point that fish oil supplements may not be good for babies and small children.

Displacement of arachidonic acid. Since the brain needs more DHA, not EPA, fish oil consumption leads to excess intake of EPA. Since excess levels of EPA can displace the critical fat, arachidonic acid, from cell membranes (and can retard infant growth), EPA is not, really, recommended for children.

Increased hemorrhage risk. As pointed out recently in several research papers, since premature babies have a high risk for brain hemorrhage they shouldn't be given an EPA-containing oil—since EPA is said to increase "bleeding time," or to decrease coagulation time, depending on how you look at it.

Infants, small children, and older adults

Depressed immune function. There are also indications that the high EPA levels in "fish oil," and in blanket-omega–3 supplements could suppress immunity in vulnerable populations, such as infants, small children, and adults as they get older.

As reported in the USDA's own publication, *Agricultural Research,* in 1990, Simin Meydani, Ph.D., a researcher at the USDA's Human Nutrition Research Center on Aging at Tufts University, in Boston, found that when older women took fish oil capsules, certain immune-function markers—cytokines—were suppressed.

In fact, the EPA-rich fish oil supplements also put a "wet blanket" on the immune system's response to an experimentally produced infection. The fish oil reduced cytokine production by *63 percent!* This is important, especially since the cytokine in question is involved in increasing the number of T cells that can be mobilized against "foreign invaders."

This led Meydani to say that "the beneficial anti-inflammatory effect of fish oil must be weighed against its effect on T-cell-mediated immune response, especially in older women." In other words, of course, fish oil has its benefits, but its drawbacks, as well.

Let's look at the benefits.

The benefits

Although fish oil's heart-friendly effects had been noted as early as 1956 (Bronte-Stewart, et al., *Lancet* I:521), it really took the impact of Bang and Dyerberg's groundbreaking studies of the diet of Greenland Eskimos to put fish oil omega–3 fatty acids and cardiovascular health together on the same map, in which fish plays a very large part.

Clearly, the consumption of fish and fish oils has been associated with powerful benefits for health. In fact, in January 1998, C.M. Albert, et al., published a study in the *Journal of the American Medical Association*, which looked at fish consumption in 20,551 U.S. male physicians who participated in the U.S. Physicians' Health Study. The study concluded that "consumption of fish, at least once per week, may reduce the risk of sudden cardiac death in men." Interested?

I am—and you will be, too. And in a National Library of Medicine MEDLINE search on fish/fish oil studies that came out in 1998, I found, in part, the following:

- The omega–3 fatty acids in fish oil significantly decrease (experimentally) primary breast tumor growth and metastasis (spreading to other tissue)—[Hubbard, et al., *Cancer Letter* 124(1):1–7, 1998]
- Fish oil experimentally protects against colon cancer [W.L. Chang, et al., *Journal of Nutrition* 128(3):491–497, 1998]
- Menhaden oil experimentally prevents diet caused insulin resistance [D.A. Podolin, et al., *American Journal of Physiology* 274(3, II):R840-848, 1998]
- Whale/seal oil consumption in humans causes changes in platelet membranes and response, which help circulation [E. Vognild, et al., *Lipids* 33(4):427–436, 1998]

Nevertheless, some surprises do crop up with full-spectrum fish oil supplementation, such as unexpected *increases* in low-density-lipoprotein (LDL), or "bad" cholesterol and immune suppression—on the one hand—with cancer-protection on the other, as noted in Friedberg's article in *Diabetes Care*.

We'll get to the most serious problem in a minute, but first, let's take a brief look at **snake oil** (yes, snake oil).

Snake Oil

Dr. Udo Erasmus opened my eyes to the potential health benefits of this most maligned of "medicines." Although many of us think of the nostrums and elixirs dispensed by those itinerant "Traveling Medicine Show" hucksters of yore, or "Snake-Oil Salesmen" as they were called, actual snake oil (in jar or bottle form for topical use) originated in China, where it was rubbed on to reduce pain and swelling in rheumatoid arthritis and other inflammatory conditions, such as bursitis.

According to Erasmus, a California doctor took snake oil that he picked up in San Francisco's Chinatown and had it analyzed. Aside from a carrier fluid and camphor, 25 percent of the snake oil product was derived apparently, from Chinese water snakes; 20 percent of the product contained the anti-inflammatory fatty acid, EPA, which can be absorbed through the skin.

I guess we'd better come up for a more disparaging name for those old-time bamboozlers, since it seems that "snake-oil salesman" can now be taken as a compliment!

Before we launch into the Chapter 2 overview of the research that's out there on our "star" fatty acid, DHA, let's step aside for a minute and return to one aspect of fish oil that we'd best consider.

In addition to the varying degrees of rancidity which plague full-spectrum fish oil supplements, generally speaking (although there are several top-notch fish oil supplements out there), there is a problem even more serious than that: **toxic contamination**.

Toxic contamination of fish and full-spectrum fish oil

On March 17, 1998, the radio program, *Arctic Science Journeys* began like this:

High in the Arctic, hundreds of miles north of Alaska—almost but not quite near the North Pole—you'd expect to see a stark white landscape set against a brilliant blue sky. But, instead, a layer of soot hangs in the air.

Climatologists, and other experts, call this gray layer "Arctic Haze." It seems that winds carry soot from coal burning plants and factories in Eastern Europe and Russia into the Arctic. Unfortunately, along with the soot, the winds also transport contaminants, such as mercury and lead, into the far north.

Harold Welch, a research scientist with Canada's Department of Fisheries and Oceans, describes a horrific picture. Contaminants—like DDT, toxophene, and PCBs—have made their way into the high-Arctic food chain.

Said Welch on the program, which was entitled "Top of the World Pollution" (and was narrated by Robert Hannon):

The upper 200 meters of the Arctic Ocean is the biggest reservoir, I think in the world, for these [toxic] materials. You have to understand that these pesticides evaporate quickly. So, if you spray them on a field in India, for example, they [. . .] are transported by the atmosphere to the Pole. [. . .] That's one of the ways they grasshopper their way into the Arctic Ocean.

Scary indeed. In fact, on June 7, 1995, the environmental organization, Greenpeace, issued an independently conducted analysis of 22 brands of fish oil.

In fish oil samples obtained from Norway, Japan, England, Iceland, and Germany, 21 of the 22 brands were found to contain high levels of hazardous contaminants, specifically the organochlorine pesticides, DDT and lindane, and PCBs. The report said that: "Anyone taking a therapeutic dose would reach 80% of the U.S. FDA-mandated maximum levels for these pollutants"!

The nightmare looks like this: Toxic chemicals enter bodies of water from industrial dumping in rivers and runoff from contaminated land. These pollutants are then carried by oceanic and atmospheric currents to remote ocean regions like the Arctic. Fish pick up the toxins via the food chain (zooplankton, for example), and their livers concentrate the poisonous residues.

Not the prettiest of pictures. So how can we reap the benefits of omega–3 sources without risking any, or all, of the aforementioned problems?

Enter **DHA**.

Do All Roads to Health "Stop at" DHA?

In many ways, yes. Although DHA is only one "panel" in an ever-evolving nutritional tapestry, this panel is crucial to the whole design. Natural DHA oil is extracted—and purified—from ocean-dwelling, single-cell microalgae.

The main structural fat of both the brain and retina, DHA is an omega–3 fat that is not only critically important but, truly is: *essential for life.*

References

Aro, A., et al. "Adipose tissue isomeric *trans* fatty acids and risk of myocardial infarction in nine countries: the EURAMIC study," *Lancet* 345:273–278, 1995.

Albert, C.M., et al. "Fish consumption and risk of sudden cardiac death." *Journal of the American Medical Association* 279(1):23–28, 1998.

Bang, H.O., et al. "The composition of food consumed by Greenlandic Eskimos," *Acta Med Scand* 200:69–73, 1973.

Bronte-Stewart, B., et al. "Effects of feeding different fats on serum cholesterol levels," *Lancet* I:521, 1956.

Chow, C.K. *Fatty Acids in Foods and Their Health Implications.* New York: Marcel Dekker, 1992.

Connor, William E., et al. "N–3 fatty acids from fish oil: effects on plasma lipoproteins and hypertriglyceridemic patients," *Journal of the New York Academy of Sciences* 683:16–34, 1993.

Dyerberg, J., and Bang, H.O. "Hemostatic function and platelet polyunsaturated fatty acids in Eskimos," *Lancet* 433–435, 1979.

Enig, Mary G. "Trans fatty acids: an update," *Nutrition Quarterly* 17(4):79–95, 1993.

Enig, Mary. "Isomeric trans fatty acids in the U.S. diet," *Journal of the American College of Nutrition* 9(5):471–486.

Erasmus, Udo, Ph.D. *Fats That Heal, Fats That Kill.* Burnaby, B.C., Canada: Alive Books, 1993.

Friedberg, C.E., et al. "Fish oil and glycemic control in diabetes: a meta-analysis." *Diabetes Care* 21(4):494–500, 1998.

Gormley, James J., and Scheer, James F. "Fats—a rational approach," *Better Nutrition* 60 (3): 52–58, 1998.

Gormley, James J. "Fats: The Good, the Bad, and the Ugly: Moving Away From Fat Paranoia." Address given at the First Annual "Hudson Valley Health, Fitness & Nutrition Expo," Kingston, New York, November 1, 1997.

Guest, Donna K. "Test Yourself: Fats," *Better Nutrition* 59 (12):58, 1997.

Leveille, Gilbert A., Ph.D., and Mark Dreher, Ph.D. "Dietary Fat and Health," *Nutrition & the M.D.* 24(5), May 1998.

Litin, L., and Sacks, S. "Trans-fatty-acid content of common foods," *New England Journal of Medicine* 329(26), 1996.

Mensink, R.P., and Katan, M.B. "Effect of dietary *trans* fatty acids on high-density and low-density lipoprotein cholesterol levels in healthy subjects," *New England Journal of Medicine* 323:439–445, 1990.

Simopoulos, Artemis P., M.D., and Robinson, Jo. *The Omega Plan: The Medically Proven Diet That Restores Your Body's Essential Nutritional Balance.* New York: HarperCollins, 1998.

Watt, Bernice K., and Merrill, Annabel L. *Composition of Foods: Raw, Processed, Prepared.* Agriculture Handbook No. 8. Washington, D.C.: USDA Agricultural Research Service, October 1975. Catalog number: A1.76:8/963.

Willett, Walter C., M.D., et al. *"Trans-*fatty acid intake in relation to risk of coronary heart disease among women," *Lancet* 341:581–585, 1993.

CHAPTER 2

DHA—what the research is telling us

The world wants to be deceived.

Narrenschiff, c. 1494

Yes, we have been deceived about the true story of fats. But let's step back a bit, and see what happened. Since the 1960s, science has been uncovering the science behind the good fats, what the prenatal and infant brain needs for the right structure and development, and what balance of good fats children and adults need throughout their lives.

As we saw in the last chapter, the U.S. food industry's exclusive love affair with polyunsaturated fatty acids from land vegetables is over. We've looked at how top-heavy the American diet has been with low-end (partially hydrogenated) omega–6 fatty acids and how dangerously low it's been in omega–3 fatty acids (including DHA).

The Good News, the Bad News, and Some Problems

The good news is that our evolutionary ancestors didn't have a problem with an imbalance of omega–6 fats compared to omega–3 fats—their ratio was close to 1:1 (some experts say 2½:1). The bad news is that *we do* have a problem. The typical U.S. diet has a profile of anywhere from 10:1 to 22:1, omega–6 to omega–3 fats.

As we've discovered, while some of the omega–6-heavy oils are very nutritious—such as hemp, evening primrose, black currant seed, and borage seed—it's a disappointment, but no surprise, that the most nutritionally imbalanced of the omega–6 oils, those with the highest amounts of artery-clogging saturated fats, for example, are the oils most used in mass market foods: coconut oil and palm oil.

There are also vegetable oils that have good omega–3-acid profiles: flax seed, canola, and pumpkin seed and those which are high in omega–3-"propagating" linolenic acid: sunflower oil and sesame oil, for example.

As we've seen, most Americans are taking in highly processed oils with the highest saturated fat content, oils that have been extracted with chemicals, hydrogenated, bleached, heated to high temperatures, "purified," and turned into stick margarine. Adding insult to injury, the very process of hydrogenation itself transforms the molecular structure of these fats into harmful, unnatural forms.

The Push to Eat Low Fat

Well, it was more of a shove than a push. Over the past 50 years, the government and the mass-market food industry have shifted the American diet away from eggs, lard, and organ meats, and toward foods dominated by highly processed omega–6-rich land-vegetable oils, as we saw above.

This downward spiral in the omega–3-fat consumption of the typical American diet has reverse-paralleled the dizzying upward spiral in the number of research papers that have come out in the past 30 years documenting the critical value of sufficient—better yet, optimal—intake of key omega–3 fatty acids, including: docosapentaenoic acid (DPA), eicosapentaenoic acid (EPA), and docosahexaenoic acid (DHA).

What's a DHA and Where Do I Get It?

DHA is the primary structural fatty acid in the brain and in the retina (Figure 2–1). We get DHA in our diets, first through the placenta before birth, then through breast milk, then through such dietary sources as fish (cod, tuna, salmon, and sardines), red meat, animal organ meats, and eggs, as mentioned.

Since our bodies make such a small quantity of this essential fat, we have to look to dietary sources and supplementation to meet our needs. Vegetarians, in particular, have even lower blood levels of DHA because it's practically absent from most land-based, or terrestrial, plants.

Is adding fish oil supplements to our diet enough? Not quite. While there are some excellent fish oil supplements available in health food stores, DHA is a fatty acid perfectly suited for taking as a single nutrient. In its capsule form, for instance, manufacturers are able to concentrate the level of DHA for specific needs and groups, such as for pregnant and lactating women, whose omega–3 needs are higher than those of other people.

If fish oil isn't the final answer here, then what is? To find out, let's take a closer look at what goes on in the ocean food chain. In fact, let's focus on the most populous living creature in the sea, the phytoplankton, a major source of fish food. Phytoplankton are ocean dwelling microalgae concentrated in omega–3 fatty acids. The more they eat, the more omega–3 fatty acids

What is DHA?

DHA is an unusual fatty acid which is highly unsaturated (C22:6), and is an integral component of membranes with electrical activity (e.g., neurons, retina, heart, etc.).

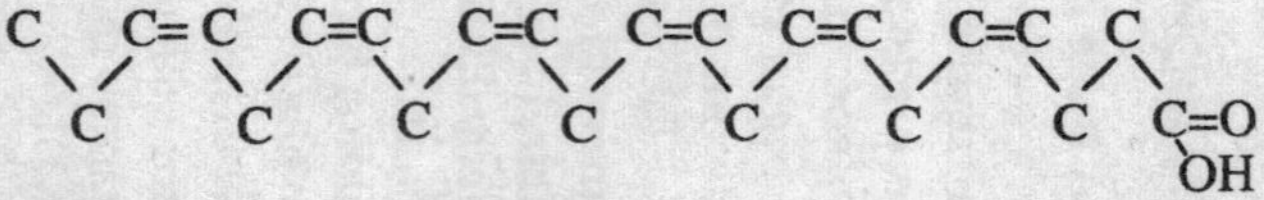

Figure 2-1

they consume. Unfortunately, since we know that fish oils can come with toxins and chemical pollutants picked up in our trash-filled waters, one way of ensuring that an uncompromised source of DHA is available to us comes by purifying it from these microalgae to preset concentrations (See the Appendix for more information).

The Research and this Book

In Parts II, III, IV, and V, we'll be looking, in depth, at much of the research on DHA and speaking with some of the scientists who've carried out the studies; there will also be a testimonial from a mother whose child suffered from Attention Deficit Disorder, and her boy's success at finding a cure with DHA.

Before there were successes, of course, there was the research. One of the earliest modern studies of fats and nutrition appeared in 1930, when G.O. Burr and M.M. Burr published a landmark study of essential fatty acids: "On the Nature of the Fatty Acids Essential in Nutrition," a paper which, in part, established the nutritional importance of the omega–6, linoleic acid, and its breakdown fat, arachidonic acid, both critical to growth and development.

Unfortunately, it's the omega–3s (especially DHA) in which the typical Western diet is embarrassingly lacking (Figures 2–2 and 2–3).

The Newest Understanding of Fatty Acids and DHA

Major news conference in New York City

On April 3, 1997, a groundbreaking conference was held at New York Hospital-Cornell Medical Center. It

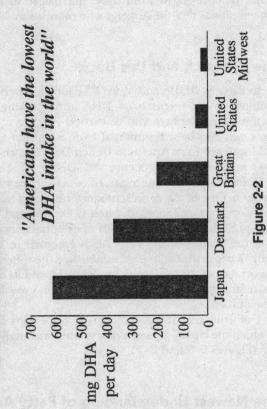

DHA Intake

"Americans have the lowest
DHA intake in the world"

mg DHA
per day

700
600
500
400
300
200
100
0

Japan   Denmark   Great Britain   United States   United States Midwest

Figure 2-2

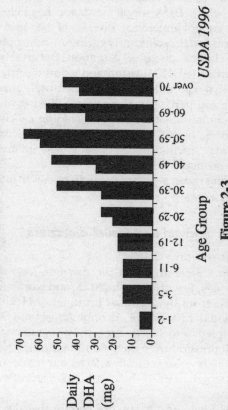

Present DHA Consumption in the United States

Daily DHA (mg)

Age Group

1-2 3-5 6-11 12-19 20-29 30-39 40-49 50-59 60-69 over 70

USDA 1996

Figure 2-3

was entitled "Keeping Your Brain In Shape: New Insights Into DHA," which I discussed in my June 1997 *Better Nutrition* editorial: "DHA and the Excitement of New Research."

At the news conference, some of the areas covered with which DHA supplementation has helped include (but are not limited to): diseases of the mind (including depression, hostility and aggression, schizophrenia, and Alzheimer's disease); Attention Deficit Hyperactivity Disorder (ADHD); vision and vision disorders (including dyslexia and retinitis pigmentosa); specific metabolic and peroxisomal disorders; diseases of immunity, inflammation, and allergy (including cancer, multiple sclerosis, or MS, inflammatory bowel disease, or IBD, asthma); cardiovascular health; and infants' prenatal and postnatal development.

Let's take a glance now at research into some of these areas.

Neurological and visual disorders

Depression

In a 1995 article in the *American Journal of Clinical Nutrition,* Joseph Hibbeln, M.D., and Norman Salem, Jr., Ph.D., from the National Institutes of Health's (NIHs) National Institute of Alcohol Abuse and Alcoholism, grappled with North America's documented increase in depression over the past 100 years, a period of time in which we've radically altered our intake of fats from that which marked the past 12,000 years of evolutionary history.

Hibbeln and Salem are certain that the decreasing omega–3 levels in the typical U.S. diet "may also affect the nervous system, in early development or adulthood," increasing our chances of developing depression.

Societies which regularly chow down on omega–3-

rich fish—such as Taiwan, Hong Kong, mainland China, and Japan—have much lower rates of depression than we do in North America: 10 times lower, in fact, if we take Taiwan as the comparison point.

Recognizing the possible relationship between lowered rates of depression and level of omega–3 intake, Hibbeln and Salem also cite the issue of cholesterol. In fact, they specifically criticize the belief that lowered cholesterol will help to solve the problem of depression. "The endpoint of serum cholesterol may not be specific enough," they say, pointing to other recent studies showing increased depression and increased risk of coronary artery disease associated with a general decrease in dietary fats.

Even further, they point to a more troubling fact— the "party line" about fats in the diet overly encouraging patients to consume foods with yet higher levels of low-end omega–6 fatty acids, leading to DHA *deficiency*. It is a problem associated with such conditions as alcoholism and multiple sclerosis, and to the depression which often accompanies them.

In a July 1998 interview, Hibbeln makes it doubly clear that he doesn't buy into the party line on fats.

Hostility and aggression

Hibbeln's works crop up again in reference to hostility, mainly because there may be a nutritional imbalance commonality linked to both depression and what are called "type-A" measures of hostility.

According to Hibbeln, a number of studies have "suggested that violent, impulsive prisoners appear to be deficient in [DHA]," compared to control subjects on similar diets. He added that: "[DHA] supplementation reduced aggression in Japanese students, who already have high levels of omega–3 fats" in their diets.

In this regard, Hibbeln suggests that we look at how

DHA, and other omega–3 fatty acids, may be related to low levels of another brain neurotransmitter, serotonin.

Hibbeln goes on to conclude that recent studies "which have suggested that cholesterol-lowering diets may increase mortality due to increased suicide and traumatic death" are significant enough to follow up with more conclusive research. At the same time, he recognizes the importance of getting optimal levels of DHA and other omega–3 fats into those who have been diagnosed as depressive and/or hostile-aggressive, including those who are institutionalized.

Multiple Sclerosis (MS)

In 1990, D. Bates linked high levels of depression with patients with MS, showing that fatty acid supplements improve both quality-of-life and physical symptoms.

Schizophrenia

The medical journal, *Schizophrenia Research*, published a study in 1994 which examined levels of saturated fatty acids and long-chain omega–3 fatty acids in red blood cell (RBC) membranes of 68 subjects with schizophrenia and 259 subjects without.

The researchers, led by A.I.M. Glen of Inverness, Scotland's Highland Psychiatric Research Group, found that a "subgroup of schizophrenics have abnormally low" levels of the omega–3 fatty acids in RBC membranes, which extends earlier findings of K.S. Vaddadi, published in 1985 and 1992.

Glen was also quite clear as to the implications involved here. "If our finding applies to other membranes, the proposed developmental abnormality in some schizophrenic patients might be explained by a [deficiency] of membrane fatty acids," he concluded.

Are Glen's findings exciting? You bet; and for two

immediate reasons. First, because the abnormalities reported in dopamine levels, for example, which have been part of the main focus of biochemical-based research into schizophrenia, may be less critical than the levels of good fats in cell membranes.

Second, new ways of specifically looking at, and nutritionally treating, those people with schizophrenia who don't show any of the usually negative symptoms associated with the disease are now available.

Exciting research also is uncovering links between DHA-supplementation and protection against alcohol caused damage, much of the research for which has been carried out by N. Salem, Ph.D.

Alzheimer's Disease

We know that the body produces DHA, but it does so in insufficient amounts. For example, while the body does produce some DHA from alpha linolenic acid, as Ernst J. Schaefer, M.D., chief of the Lipid Metabolism Laboratory at Tufts University's Human Nutrition Research Center on Aging, explains: "Humans, particularly infants and the elderly, who produce it even less efficiently, rely on their diets for DHA from sources such as fish."

Although plasma DHA levels are relatively low normally (yet concentrated in the brain and retina), Schaefer and colleagues decided to go ahead and measure plasma DHA levels in 1,137 patients to see if those with senile dementia, including Alzheimer's disease, had even lower levels.

They found that people who were in the "low DHA" group were about 1.7 times more likely to develop dementia, leading Schaefer to note that "decreased DHA content is associated with an increased risk of developing dementia, including Alzheimer's disease."

Attention deficit hyperactivity disorder (ADHD)

Purdue University's John R. Burgess, Ph.D., has also pursued lines of research that bear some relevance to the relationship between DHA levels in the body and ADHD. As he wrote: "Studies have indicated that children with ADHD report symptoms that are similar to those observed in essential fatty acid (EFA) deficiency in both animals and humans deprived of EFA."

Burgess took these findings to the next logical step, suggesting that some children with ADHD could have a malfunctioning mechanism which stores, mobilizes, and breaks down fatty acids.

In another study by Laura J. Stevens, Ph.D., which appeared in the *American Journal of Clinical Nutrition* in 1995, a subgroup of young patients with ADHD who reported many symptoms that usually tell of a lack of the good fats (EFA deficiencies) also "had significantly lower blood plasma levels" of DHA and arachidonic acid than did children with ADHD who only had a few symptoms of EFA deficiency.

In 1996, Stevens took another look at the data from the 1995 study. She and her colleagues confirmed that children with "lower omega–3 fatty acid levels showed a significantly greater number of behavior problems."

Her conclusion was summed up this way by collaborator, Burgess: "In the brain, a sub-clinical deficiency of DHA may be responsible for the abnormal behavior of these children." In truth, it's not only children who are affected by ADHD. Some recent estimates suggest that between 6 to 9.5 million American adults have the disorder, as well.

In Chapter 4, we will talk with a mother, whom we will call Lola, who will tell us of her results with DHA and attention deficit hyperactivity disorder (ADHD) in her son, whom we shall call Justin—a truly wonderful, and true, story.

Vision disorders

Since, as we have seen, levels of DHA in the retina and brain are supposed to be highly concentrated, it's not surprising that a metabolic "monkey wrench" gives rise to very low levels of this fatty acid, the understanding of which has been accumulating over the past 14 years, and which is now associated with conditions as different as **dyslexia** and **retinitis pigmentosa**.

In 1995, researchers Dennis R. Hoffman, Ph.D., and David G. Birch, Ph.D., from Texas' Retina Foundation of the Southwest, measured fatty acid levels in the red blood cells of patients with what is called X-linked retinitis pigmentosa (XLRP, or RP), the most serious genetic kind of retinitis pigmentosa, a hereditary degenerative disease marked, in part, by night blindness and loss of peripheral vision.

The fact is that the total level of fatty acids is supposed to reach levels of 30 to 40 percent in "rod photoreceptor" portions of the human retina, forming the basis for an important relationship between retinal function and red blood cell DHA levels.

Their findings led them to conclude that: "Dietary supplementation [with] DHA would bypass several of the [steps] and may restore blood levels of DHA to normal, regardless of the specific mechanism" which is not functioning correctly.

They went on to say that we now must think about "the potential for early nutritional intervention to delay the degenerative rod loss in patients" with this problem.

Genetic/metabolic disorders

Sometimes people are born with real problems in how their bodies deal with fat, specifically in how they break it down, assemble its molecules, and so on. These uncommon disorders are often tragic in the physical suffering and hardship they bring, often to infants and small children. Thus, our focus, for the moment at least, will be on Zellweger's syndrome. In Chapter 8, I will broaden this discussion to include related diseases such as Pseudo-Zellweger syndrome, Juvenile Neuronal Ceroid-Lipofuscinosis (JNCL), also called Batten's disease, and phenylketonuria (PKU), also called Folling's disease.

Zellweger's syndrome

Zellweger's syndrome has been called the "proto-type of generalized peroxisomal disorders," liver peroxisomes being nearly absent in the most serious cases.

The syndrome is a fatal genetic disease, one which ushers in severe neurological symptoms from birth, such as seizures, compromised mental control of voluntary movement, and visual impairment. Death usually occurs before 6 months of age, preceded by serious abnormalities having to do with peripheral nerves, including breakdown of the protein/fat sheaths which protect nerve fibers, called myelin.

In a chapter written by Manuela Martinez, Ph.D., of Spain's Autonomous University of Barcelona, which appeared in the volume, *Health Effects of Omega–3 Polyunsaturated Fatty Acids in Seafoods* in 1991, it was said that "the most important abnormality was a significant decrease in the brain levels of [DHA]" compared with normal ranges. The liver levels of DHA were extremely low, "virtually negligible," in most of the cases reviewed.

Martinez also recommended that a DHA-rich diet be given (under supervision) to "peroxisomal patients."

I would go one step further and suggest that scientists and clinicians consider a DHA-boosted diet for pregnant and breastfeeding women, and addition of omega–3 fatty acids to infant formula as prudent steps that could only help.

Diseases of Immunity, Inflammation, and the Heart

In further chapters, we'll show how DHA and these vectors converge as we move from the cancer research of M. Noguchi (1995) and Gogos (1998), to multiple sclerosis (MS) and the researches of Bates and Nightingale (1990), to rheumatoid arthritis and Joel Kremer (1995), to asthma and other allergic conditions as researched by Black and Sharpe (1997) and Broughton (1997), to inflammatory bowel disease (Stenson, 1995), to diseases of the heart.

The DHA/cardiovascular research ranges from a 1988 study by Gregory Dehmer, M.D., to 1998 research by Michael Miller, M.D., and paints quite a fascinating picture, one that has largely been ignored by many.

Infant nutrition

The human brain is 60 percent structural fat, which uses DHA and arachidonic acid for "growth, function and integrity," said researcher Michael Crawford, Ph.D., in 1993.

The experimental evidence, which continues to build up, is that fatty acid deficiencies during early brain and neural development cause serious problems that are devastating to health and well-being and usually permanent.

Low-birth-weight babies, including very-low-birthweight and premature babies, are at the highest risk of what are called neurodevelopmental disorders, including cerebral palsy. Other areas that are affected by such disorders include: intelligence quotients and cognitive ability; vision and peripheral neuropathy; and an increased risk (on the part of the baby) for developing noninsulin-dependent diabetes and vascular disease in later life

In 1994, the World Health Organization issued its "Food and Nutrition Paper No. 57." The policy paper concluded, in part, that "it would seem proper to provide both arachidonic acid and DHA preformed [as single nutrient or joint nutrient supplements] in term infant formula milks in similar proportions to breast milk from well-nourished, omnivorous mothers."

We'll also unveil an 18-year study that appeared in the journal, *Pediatrics*, and which found that the DHA in breast milk helps to increase I.Q. and later educational achievement—pretty groundbreaking findings!

According to David Kyle, Ph.D., senior vice president for research and development at Maryland-based Martek Biosciences, "medical experts consider DHA an essential nutrient in the diets of infants" because of the rapid brain growth that occurs at this early stage of life.

A New Paradigm in Nutrition?

So there you have it—the briefest of overviews for an exciting, yet daunting, collection of the world's research into DHA, docosahexaenoic acid, the nutritional gem of the long-chain omega–3 fatty acids.

Kyle believes that science is on the verge of understanding a new paradigm in nutrition. While the importance of certain vitamins, minerals and amino acids "that make up the structure of our body is known, [. . .] now researchers are beginning to understand the importance of the essential fats"—the Good Fats!

Let's get started.

References

Bates, D. "Dietary lipids and multiple sclerosis," *Uppsala Journal of Medical Science* S48: 173–187, 1990.

Burr, G.O., and Burr, M.M. "On the Nature of the Fatty Acids Essential in Nutrition," *Journal of Biology and Chemistry* 86: 587–621, 1930.

Colquhoun, I., and Bunday, S. "A Lack of Essential Fatty Acids as a Possible Cause of Hyperactivity in Children," *Medical Hypotheses* 673–679, 1981.

Crawford, Michael A. "The role of essential fatty acids in neural development: implications for perinatal nutrition," *American Journal of Clinical Nutrition* 57:703S–710S, 1993.

Crawford, M.A., et al. "Omega–6 and omega–3 fatty acids during early development," *Journal of Internal Medicine* 225:159–169, 1989.

Dobbing, J. "Vulnerable Periods in Brain Development." In: K. Elliott and E. Knight (editors): *Lipids, Malnutrition & the Developing Brain.* Amsterdam: Associated Scientific Publishers, 1972, pp. 9–29.

FAO/WHO Expert Committee. "Food and Nutrition Paper No. 57." In: *Fats and Oils in Human Nutrition,* 1994, pp. 49–55.

Gerstl, B., et al. "Alterations in Myelin Fatty Acids and Plasmalogens in Multiple Sclerosis," *Annals of the New York Academy of Sciences* 122: 405–407, 1965.

Glen, A.I.M., et al. "A Red Cell Abnormality in a Subgroup of Schizophrenic Patients: Evidence for Two Diseases," *Schizophrenia Research* 12: 53–61, 1994.

Hibbeln, Joseph R., Ph.D., and Salem, Norman, Jr., Ph.D. "Dietary Polyunsaturated Fatty Acids and Depression: When Cholesterol Does Not Satisfy," *American Journal of Clinical Nutrition* 62: 1–9, 1995.

Hoffman, Dennis R., Ph.D., and Birch, David G., Ph.D. "Docosahexaenoic Acid in Red Blood Cells of Patients With X-Linked Retinitis Pigmentosa," *Investigative Ophthalmology & Visual Science* 36 (6): 1009–1018, May 1995.

Holman, Ralph T., Ph.D., et al. "Deficiencies of Polyun-saturated Fatty Acids and Replacement by Nonessential Fatty Acids in Plasma Lipids in Multiple Sclerosis," *Proceedings of the National Academy of Sciences of the United States of America* 86: 4720–4724, June 1989.

Horwood, L. John, M.Sc., and Fergusson, David M., Ph.D. "Breastfeeding and later cognitive and academic outcomes," *Pediatrics* 101(1):1–7, 1998.

Martinez, Manuela, Ph.D. "Developmental Profiles of Polyunsaturated Fatty Acids in the Brain of Normal Infants and Patients With Peroxisomal Diseases: Severe Deficiency of Docosahexaenoic Acid in Zellweger's and Pseudo-Zellweger's Syndromes." In: Simopoulos, A. P., et al. (editors): *Health Effects of Omega–3 Polyunsaturated Fatty Acids in Seafoods* (Series: *World Review of Nutrition and Dietetics*), 66: 87–102, 1991.

Nightingale, S., et al. "Red Blood Cell and Adipose Tissue Fatty Acids in Mild Inactive Multiple Sclerosis," *Acta Neurologica Scandinavica* 82: 43–50, 1990.

Olegard, R., and Svennerholm, L. "Fatty Acid Composi-tion of Plasma and Red Cell Phosphoglycerides in Full-Term Infants and Their Mothers," *Acta Paediatrica Scandinavica* 59: 637–647, 1970.

Schaefer, Ernst J., M.D. "Decreased plasma phosphati-dylcholine docosahexaenoic acid content in dementia." Presented at: Keeping Your Brain in Shape—New Insights into DHA, New York City, April 3, 1997.

Stevens, Laura J., Ph.D., *et al.* "Essential Fatty Acid Metabolism in Boys With Attention Deficit Hyperactivity Disorder," *American Journal of Clinical Nutrition* 62: 761–768, 1995.

PART II

▼

DHA— Neurological and Visual Disorders

"If we consider the history of evolution, it is evident that the very earliest development of photoreceptors, nervous systems and brains were associated with [the] dominant availability of omega–3 fatty acids, and it so happens that we now know that both photoreceptors and synaptic junctions use a preponderance of the omega–3 fatty acids," said Michael A. Crawford in his landmark 1990 review article, "The Early Development and Evolution of the Human Brain."

In other words, the eyes and brain use a lot of omega–3 fats, especially DHA. In fact, as we've already seen, DHA is the building block of the human brain. With up to 60 percent of the brain composed of fat, DHA is the most abundant single fat in both the brain and the retina.

In truth, DHA is the "major polyunsaturated fatty acid (PUFA) in the central nervous system (CNS)," according to Norman Salem, Ph.D., chief of the NIH's Laboratory of Membrane Biochemistry and Biophysics at the National Institute of Alcohol Abuse and Alcoholism (NIAAA).

Exciting links between levels of DHA and seemingly unrelated neurological and behavioral conditions have been uncovered (Figure 3-1), including: Alzheimer's disease; depression, hostility, and aggression; attention deficit hyperactivity disorder (ADHD); metabolic and peroxisomal disorders; and vision.

Interestingly enough, only relatively small increases in diet, and dietary-supplement, levels of DHA are often enough to effect profound improvements in health.

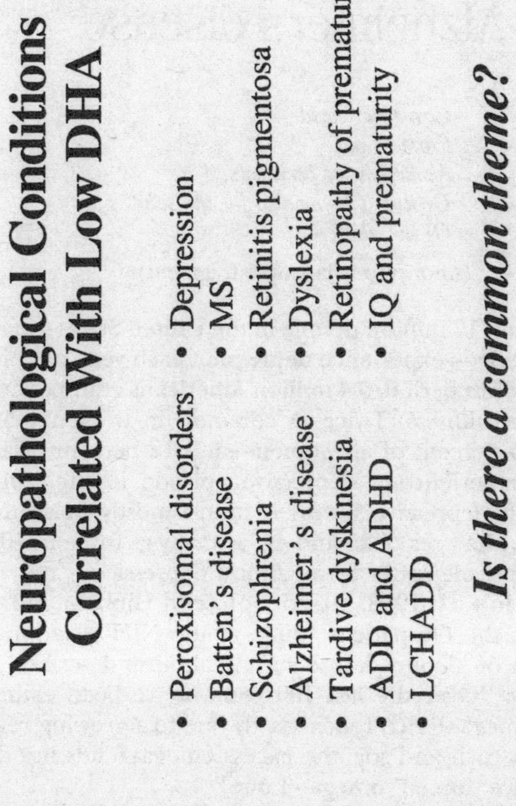

Neuropathological Conditions Correlated With Low DHA

- Peroxisomal disorders
- Batten's disease
- Schizophrenia
- Alzheimer's disease
- Tardive dyskinesia
- ADD and ADHD
- LCHADD

- Depression
- MS
- Retinitis pigmentosa
- Dyslexia
- Retinopathy of prematurity
- IQ and prematurity

Is there a common theme?

Figure 3-1

CHAPTER 3

··

Diseases of the mind: depression, schizophrenia, and Alzheimer's disease

Can this world
From of old
Always have been so sad,
Or did it become so for the sake
Of me alone

(Anonymous Japanese fragment)

More than 17 million people in the United States—one in 10 adults—experience **depression** each year, and, in any 6-month period, 9.4 million Americans grapple with depressive illness. Twice as common in women than men, 25 percent of all women—and 12 percent of all men—experience a depressive episode in life. And although depressive illness is found mostly in adults between the ages of 25 and 44, as many as three in 100 elderly people suffer from clinical depression.

In a July 21, 1998, interview, Joseph Hibbeln, M.D., chief of the Outpatient Clinic at the NIH's National Institute of Alcohol Abuse and Alcoholism described it this way: "Over the last 100 years, we've been eating more omega–6-rich foods, partly due to a growing reliance on corn and soy; the excess omega–6 fats in our diets have 'forced' omega–3 out."

This "force out" clearly helps no one, much less those individuals who are most vulnerable to the ravages of widespread essential fatty acid deficiency, including

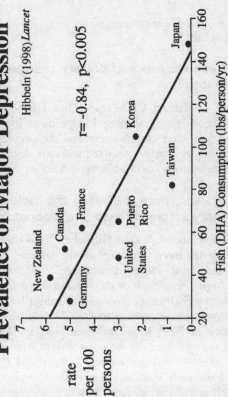

DHA Consumption Predicts Prevalence of Major Depression

Hibbeln (1998) *Lancet*

r= -0.84, p<0.005

rate per 100 persons

Fish (DHA) Consumption (lbs/person/yr)

Figure 3-2

those suffering with diseases of the mind, such as depression and **schizophrenia**. In this light, depression and other like disorders have been linked to low DHA consumption (Figures 3–1 and 3–2).

First let's take a look at depression.

Depression

Have these widespread dietary changes been documented?

"Yes," explained DHA researcher Hibbeln. "The changes in our national diet, along with an increase in saturated fats, have clearly increased the prevalence of coronary artery disease, which has been documented by the Epidemiological Catchment Area survey."

Is there a link, then, between the incidence of coronary artery disease and depression?

"It's well known," said Hibbeln, "that depression predicts death from coronary artery disease, and that the two have been closely associated."

The high prevalence of depression in patients with coronary artery disease, alcoholism, multiple sclerosis, and postpartum depression may all be tied to low concentrations of DHA in neural membranes. "Deficient levels of omega–3 in the nervous system may increase the vulnerability to depression," explained Hibbeln, "just as a deficient level in the circulation may increase vulnerability to heart disease."

A fish story?

A study recently conducted by Hibbeln found a 60-fold difference in the prevalence of depression in different countries, all correlated to how much fish is consumed on a per capita basis. "High fish consumption was associated with a low prevalence of depression," Hibbeln pointed out.

In fact, in cross-national studies comparing diets, researchers have found that in countries where fish is a main element of the diet, such as Taiwan and Japan, rates of depression were lower than in North American and European populations.

Nevertheless, it's important that we don't forget the larger "fish story" we read about in Chapter 1, where we noted the risks, and benefits, of attempting to obtain the DHA we need from fish sources alone.

How does DHA influence something like depression?

Well aside from the fact that DHA is highly concentrated in the brain, Hibbeln has observed that, in healthy patients, high levels of plasma DHA and arachidonic acid "predicted higher CSF [cerebrospinal fluid] concentrations of neurotransmitter breakdown components, 5–HIAA (from serotonin) and HVA (from dopamine)." This is important, says Hibbeln, because low levels of these compounds are predictors of impulsive or violent behavior, and suicide.

But how can this be? To find out, we must turn to **serotonin**, an organic compound (formed from tryptophan) which is especially concentrated in the brain. Involved in many areas of brain function, serotonin is also necessary for communication between nerve cells generally and for regulation of a variety of processes in the body.

Most drugs used to treat depression are designed to raise brain concentrations of serotonin. Interestingly enough the DHA and depression studies clearly "suggest that a higher intake of DHA and arachidonic acid might [also] raise brain serotonin levels," adds Hibbeln.

In another, more recent March 1998 study on the possible relationship between DHA levels and depression, researchers D. Horrobin and M. Peet looked at the fatty acid composition of red cell membranes in 15 patients with depression and 15 patients without depression. The results? They found that the depressive patients in their study showed significantly low levels of total omega–3s, which was especially true with DHA.

DHA in hostility and aggression

Studies suggest that hostility and aggression may be increased by low levels of omega–3s. Researchers have found, for example, that prisoners who are violent and impulsive are also low in omega–3s compared to "normal" control patients. It appears then that depression, impulsivity, and aggression may be linked to out-of-whack serotonin levels, levels which, as we've seen, can be modified by supplementation with DHA.

DHA, depression, and alcoholism

Again according to Hibbeln and Salem (1995), depression secondary to alcoholism is common, occurring in 16 percent to 59 percent of alcoholic patients. Alcohol is a "prooxidant," in that it causes the "oxidation" (or "rust") of fatty acids, leading to the depletion of long-chain omega–3 fats from neuronal membranes, one of the problems associated with depressive symptoms. As a result, Hibbeln and Salem suggest that "supplementation with dietary long-chain fatty acids may speed resolution of depressive symptoms in recovering alcoholics."

Depression and multiple sclerosis (MS)

Unfortunately, a lot of people with MS are clinically depressed. The incidence of depression here is so high that some researchers have speculated that it's out-of-proportion to the incidence found in patients with similar diseases. More specifically, it has been suggested that depletion of omega–3s in the central nervous system may contribute to the increased symptoms of depression. In 1990, for instance, D. Bates (1990) showed that treatment with essential fatty acid preparations generally causes a mild reduction in relapses, and an overall reported improvement in perception of "quality of life," which "may indicate a reversal of symptoms of depression."

Schizophrenia

Stedman's defines schizophrenia in these words: "Any of a group of psychotic disorders usually characterized by withdrawal from reality, illogical patterns of thinking, delusions, and hallucinations, and accompanied in varying degrees by other emotional, behavioral, or intellectual disturbances."

This is truly a daunting constellation of symptoms. Nevertheless, research has been uncovering a lot since Horrobin's pioneer 1977 study linking schizophrenia to prostaglandin/fatty acid deficiency, a lack which he predicted was due to a defect in the breakdown, or metabolism, of fatty acids.

In 1994, for instance, a study appeared in the journal, *Schizophrenia Research*, which linked "a red cell membrane abnormality" to a group of patients with schizophrenia. Not surprisingly, this red cell membrane abnormality, in fact, took the form of a significantly lower level of 20-carbon (EPA) and 22-carbon (DHA) polyunsaturated fatty acids, a deficiency seen most clearly in those patients with the more severe form of schizophrenia, sometimes called "negative schizophrenia."

The authors' finding on membrane fatty acid deficiencies may have applications to problems associated with other, related imbalances in dopamine levels, estrogen levels, and angiotensin levels, and to part of the "environment-caused" genetic changes that may, to a degree, underpin schizophrenia.

Tardive dyskinesia

Movement disorders such as tardive dyskinesia occur in patients with schizophrenia and manic depression, and are seen in up to 60 percent of people with these disorders who are receiving tranquilizers (neuroleptic drugs).

A 1989 study by K.S. Vaddadi (led by David F. Horrobin) used fatty acid supplements in psychiatric patients (mainly schizophrenics) with movement disorders, such as tardive dyskinesia. Capsules containing omega–6 fats (72 percent linoleic acid and 9 percent gamma-linolenic) were given to 48 patients, 39 of whom had schizophrenia (81.3 percent), five of whom had bipolar affective disorder, and four of whom had a recognized personality disorder.

Before supplementation, the schizophrenic patients with tardive dyskinesia showed severe abnormalities in essential fatty acid levels, especially in the levels of DHA, arachidonic acid and alpha-linolenic acid. Although the fatty acid supplementation really improved a number of indicators, the omega–6s that were given did not, of course, raise levels of omega–3s.

Nevertheless, the authors concluded that "these observations in both schizophrenics and alcoholics suggest that essential fatty acids may provide a new form of therapy in psychiatric disorders with minimal risk of adverse effects.''

Alcohol and DHA Levels

Although a discussion of DHA and alcohol could fit into several different chapters, since there are a number of alcohol overlaps with subgroups in depression and schizophrenia trials, it would be worthwhile here to take a brief look at alcohol and DHA levels.

Alcoholics, for example, are prone to many cognitive (mental) disorders, including loss of memory, inability to concentrate, and dementia.

In 1989, Norman Salem, Ph.D., then chief of the NIH's Section of Analytical Chemistry in the Laboratory of Clinical Studies (at the NIAAA) wrote:

> Many biochemical abnormalities have been associated with alcohol intoxication or chronic usage [...] One of the biochemical changes noted in both human alcoholics, and in animals exposed to alcohol, is an alteration in the lipid profile of various blood cells and organs.

In his article, Salem asked the question: Can fatty acid supplementation counter fatty acid deficiencies caused by chronic alcohol exposure? The answer is "yes," but, to what extent remains in question.

Omega–6 fats

At that time, Salem pointed out research that had been conducted using evening primrose oil (Glen, 1984), gamma-linolenic acid (Engler, 1987 and 1988), and saturated fat-rich coconut oil (John, 1980).

While these studies showed beneficial results, the evidence is clear that the omega–3 levels must be brought up, as well. Salem suggested supplementing the diet with *both* omega–3s and omega–6s, so that the brain deficiency in omega–3 DHA can be taken care of, and so that the omega–6 deficiency in peripheral tissues can be improved.

Omega–3 fats

In 1995, six years after Salem's review article came out ("Alcohol, Fatty Acids, and Diet"), he published an experimental study, along with Robert J. Pawlosky, of the Laboratory of Membrane Biochemistry and Biophysics, National Institutes of Health. The study looked at an experimental animal group fed a diet with low, but adequate, levels of essential fats. Within this group, select animals were also given an alcohol solution to drink.

In the brains of the alcohol-treated animals, the DHA levels decreased by 17 percent, with an associated increase in an undesirable unsaturated fat; in the retinas of these animals, the undesirable fat increased by 250 percent.

For humans, the implications of this study are clear enough.

Take-home Message?

Truly, our bodies have enough difficulty obtaining enough DHA from our diet. If we can avoid, or reduce, consumption of alcoholic beverages, then our brains and retinas will thank us.

Alzheimer's Disease

> *Of all the tyrannies on human kind*
> *The worst is that which persecutes the mind.*
>
> (John Dryden, c. 1687)

Americans are aging. In fact, a 1996 Yankelovich survey found that one of the greatest fears among Americans 51 years of age and older is senility. Ernst Schaefer, M.D., chief of the Lipid Metabolism Laboratory at Tufts University's Human Nutrition Research Center on Aging, has found that that a low level of DHA poses a significant risk factor for senile dementia (Figure 3–3), including Alzheimer's disease (Figure 3–4).

Schaefer has discovered, in fact, that the human body may experience a decreased ability to make DHA as it ages. "The data I have seen," Schaefer says, "suggest that DHA may be an important therapeutic modality in some age-related conditions, including Alzheimer's and heart disease."

Adam Drewnowski, Ph.D., director of the Program in Human Nutrition at the University of Michigan's School of Public Health, agrees, and goes on to say: "Current studies on nutrition and the elderly suggest that many conditions associated with aging, such as loss of appetite and forgetfulness, may be avoided if optimal nutrition is maintained through a diet including nutrients like DHA."

The Research

In a 1991 article (*Lipids*), M. Söderberg, and colleagues, from Sweden's Karolinska Institute, looked at autopsy results on levels of polyunsaturated fatty acids in aging and in Alzheimer's disease. This is what they found.

Low DHA—A Risk Factor for Senile Dementia

- DHA linked to neurological/visual function
- AD patients have reduced level of brain DHA
- AD patients were twice as prevalent (RR=2.21) in a group with low plasma PC-DHA
- Low serum PC-DHA is a risk factor (RR=1.67) for the onset of dementia
- Elderly women of ApoE(4) genotype and low plasma PC-DHA have a 4-fold risk of poor MMSE scores
- Serum PC-DHA can be controlled by dietary intervention
- DHA intervention improved 14/18 demented patients in Japan (Yazawa, 1996)

Figure 3-3

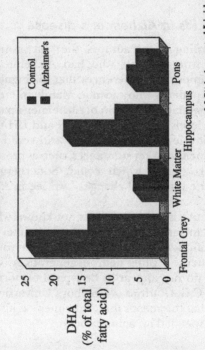

Low Brain Levels of DHA in Alzheimer's Disease

DHA
(% of total fatty acid)

25 — 20 — 15 — 10 — 5 — 0

Control
Alzheimer's

Frontal Grey   White Matter   Hippocampus   Pons

M. Söderberg, et al. Lipids (1991).

Figure 3-4

Fatty acids in aging

The samples from the non-Alzheimer's patients showed some difference from normal. While arachidonic acid levels fluctuated to a degree, the levels of DHA fluctuated considerably between normal and aging brain tissue, with levels ranging from 4 percent to 24 percent.

Fatty acids in Alzheimer's disease

According to the authors, the "fat profile" in the samples from patients who had Alzheimer's disease showed important differences that distinguish it from those of patients who did not. Mainly, there was a lot of saturated fat in the brain of Alzheimer's patients, and very low levels of arachidonic acid and DHA.

The low levels of arachidonic acid could hold back the production of key substances, such as prostaglandins and leukotrienes, which could, Söderberg suggests, "cause the functional changes" we see in Alzheimer's disease.

The authors said that "It is not known whether the changes in fatty-acid patterns in Alzheimer's patients are specific for the disease," or whether you can find these patterns in other neurodegenerative diseases. The changes do not appear to be typical of normal aging. In 1986, C.G. Gottfries of Göteborg University, Sweden, argued that this means that Alzheimer's is just an example of a speeded-up aging process.

Tin and Alzheimer's disease?

An interesting 1991 study by F.M. Corrigan and colleagues, of Argyll and Bute Hospital, U.K., "Tin and fatty acids in dementia," expands the toxic metal equation beyond aluminum, the presence of which in Alzheimer's patients has already been established.

In this study, 36 patients with senile dementia of the Alzheimer's type (SDAT), and 6 patients with multi-infarct dementia (MID), which is dementia brought on by spots of brain tissue that have "died" due to incidents of the brain's blood supply being partially cut off, were evaluated for levels of toxic metals in their bloodstream.

Dangerous levels of tin were found in the Alzheimer's patients, which is important because trimethyl tin is a neurotoxin. In animals, tin is associated with detrimental effects on copper metabolism, superoxide dismutase activity, glutathione peroxidase activity, and with harm to the good polyunsaturated fats via lipid peroxidation. DHA anyone?

PUFAs vs. Alzheimer's

In a pilot study (1996) using polyunsaturated fatty acids, Kazunaga Yazawa, Ph.D., and his colleagues from Japan's Gunma University, treated 13 people (ages 57 to 94 years) suffering from cerebrovascular dementia and 5 patients with Alzheimer's disease.

These patients received either 700 mg or 1,400 DHA in the form of "fish oil capsules." In the cerebrovascular-dementia patients, DHA yielded powerful improvements in clinical symptoms: 68.2 percent (9 of 13) "improved."

The improvements in the Alzheimer's patients were 100 percent—5 of 5 patients "slightly improved." In addition, improvement was also achieved in the following areas: communication and speech, indecisiveness, fatigue, psychological symptoms (delirium), emotional disturbance (depression), and gait (walking) disturbance.

Yazawa—who presented his findings in November 1996 at the Third Annual Conference of ISSFAL, the International Society for the Study of Fatty Acids and Lipids, in Barcelona—concluded: "These results suggest that oil rich in DHA may improve and prevent both cardiovascular dementia and Alzheimer's disease."

The phosphatidylcholine connection

DHA is actually one of two fatty acids which attaches to the brain neurotransmitter, phosphatidylcholine (PC), or, in this case PC-DHA. Ernst Schaefer of the Tufts University School of Medicine tested the hypothesis that the development of dementia, including Alzheimer's disease, is associated with decreased levels of PC-DHA.

He looked at 1,137 people who were free of dementia. Of these subjects, 64 later on developed dementia over an 8–9-year span. The incidence of new cases of dementia in the low-DHA-supplementation group was 39 out of 568, or 6.87 percent; the incidence in the high-DHA-supplementation group was 4.39 percent.

These results led Schaefer to say that "decreased plasma PC-DHA content is associated with an increasing risk of developing dementia, including Alzheimer's disease."

References

Depression: What Every Woman Should Know. Bethesda, MD: U.S. National Institutes of Health/National Institute of Mental Health. NIH Publication No. 95–3871 [no year available].

If You're 65 and Feeling Depressed. Washington, D.C.: U.S. Department of Health and Human Services. Publication No. 90–1653, 1990.

Let's Talk Facts About Depression. American Psychiatric Association. Publication No. 2252, 1994.

"What's the Best Medicine for 38 Million Mentally Ill Americans?" Mental Illness Foundation [undated].

Bates, D. "Dietary lipids and multiple sclerosis," *Uppsala Journal of Medical Sciences* S48: 173–187, 1990.

Corrigan, F.M., et al. "Tin and fatty acids in dementia," *Prostaglandins, Leukotrienes, and Essential Fatty Acids* 43:229–238, 1991.

Engler, M.M. *The Effects of Dietary Alpha- or Gamma-linolenic Acid on Fatty Acid Composition and Prostanoid Metabolism in Rat Aorta and Platelets Following Ethanol Exposure.* Washington, DC: Georgetown University; 1988. Thesis.

Engler, M.M., et al. "The effects of gamma-linolenic acid on alcohol-induced changes in fatty acid composition, blood pressure and its reactivity," *Federation Proceedings* 46:1467, 1987.

Glen, A.I.M., et al. "A Red Cell Abnormality in a Subgroup of Schizophrenic Patients: Evidence for Two Diseases," *Schizophrenia Research* 12: 53–61, 1994.

Glen, E., et al. "Possible pharmacological approaches to the prevention and treatment of alcohol related CNS impairment: Results of a double-blind trial of essential fatty acids." In: G. Edwards and J. Littleton (editors), *Pharmacological Treatments for Alcoholism.* New York: Methuen, 1984.

Gottfries, C.G. "Monoamines and myelin components in aging and dementia disorders." In: *Progress in Brain Research* 70:133–139, 1986.

Hibbeln, Joseph, and Salem, Norman, Jr. "Dietary polyunsaturated fatty acids and depression: when cholesterol does not satisfy," *American Journal of Clinical Nutrition* 62:1–9, 1995.

Peet, M., et al. "Depletion of omega–3 fatty acid levels in red-blood-cell membranes of depressive patients," *Biological Psychiatry* 43(5):315–319, 1998.

Pawlosky, Robert J., and Salem, Norman, Jr. "Ethanol exposure causes a decrease in docosahexaenoic acid and an increase in docosapentaenoic acid in feline brains and retinas," *American Journal of Clinical Nutrition* 61:1284–1289, 1995.

Salem, Norman, Jr., Ph.D. "Alcohol, Fatty Acids, and Diet," *Alcohol Health & Research World* 13(3):211–218, 1989.

Schaefer, Ernst J., M.D. "Decreased plasma phosphatidylcholine docosahexaenoic acid content in dementia." Presented at: Keeping Your Brain in Shape—New Insights into DHA, New York City, April 3, 1997.

Söderberg, M., et al. "Fatty acid composition of brain phospholipids in aging and in Alzheimer's disease," *Lipids* 26:421–425, 1991.

CHAPTER 4

....

Attention Deficit
Hyperactivity Disorder

*That energy which makes a child hard to manage is
the energy which afterward makes him a manager of life.*

Henry Ward Beecher,
Proverbs from the Plymouth Pulpit, 1887

According to the National Institute of Mental Health
(NIMH), "ADHD [. . .] is one of the most common
mental disorders [*sic*] among children. It affects 3 to 5
percent of all children, perhaps as many as 2 million
American children," and is nine-to-10 times more common in boys than in girls.

Three Main Symptoms

ADHD has three main symptoms, symptoms which
occur over a span of time: poor attention, hyperactivity,
and impulsive behavior—with ADHD itself, broken
down into "inattentive type," "hyperactive-impulsive
type," and "combined type."

According to the Florida-based group, CH.A.D.D.
(Children and Adults With Attention Deficit Disorder),
"a child may have problems listening to directions, com-
pleting assignments, or working alone without being
distracted." They continued their picture: "He [or she]
may lose things, forget things, or routinely make careless
mistakes. He [or she] may fidget, squirm, or run around

in class. He [or she] may blurt answers, interrupt, or have problems waiting his [or her] turn."

Sound like a normal, cooped-up child?

Aviva Jill Romm thinks so, who, in her 1996 book, *Natural Healing for Babies and Children,* critiques our modern, mass-market education system—a system which seems to forget that "children are naturally inclined to be energetic, physically active, and free-spirited."

McEducation?

Referred to by some as "McLearning," the children who don't fit into the Happy Meal box don't get served—they get rejected from the assembly line as "unpackageable products," Romm suggests. "If they don't fit, they must be made to. Medications create compliance, and docility in these children, and give the superficial appearance that the children *are* fitting [in], but really they are being cheated."

An "ADHD" industry?

In *No More Ritalin: Treating ADHD Without Drugs,* Mary Ann Block, D.O., P.A., offers a scalding indictment of the self-perpetuating "ADHD Industry," preferring instead to deal with the condition, as she put it so well, "without drugs" at all.

ADHD is real

True, and it's important that we remember this. So real, in fact, that John Burgess, Ph.D., assistant professor in the department of Foods and Nutrition, at Purdue University, suggests that abnormal fatty acid metabolism (Figure 4–1) may contribute to some ADHD cases.

But let's turn for a moment to a true story, this time

a success story, that I heard firsthand on July 29, 1998. On that date I interviewed the mother of a boy with ADHD—let's call her Lola—and her son, whom we can call Justin, who found relief with DHA.

JUSTIN'S STORY

LOLA: We tried Ritalin almost immediately upon diagnosis [of ADD], and there was a huge change in his behavior, for the better.

But he was unable to sleep, and he lost his appetite, and we kept him on it for about a week. And I was giving him a very low dose—I think I was giving him 5 mg/day. And he was a pretty "hyper" kid to begin with, so it didn't take much to get him over that line.

And even though he was taking it early in the morning, right before going to school, he was still not sleeping at night—he actually was externally very calm, much more calm than usual, much more focused than usual—you know, it [Ritalin] really did do what was promised—but he wasn't eating, and he wasn't sleeping.

And those are two things that you can't sacrifice. And there has to be a better solution.

It could be the "drug of choice" for that particular problem, but its side effects were not worth it, for our family at least. Justin's a very thin kid to begin with, and I can't afford to have him lose weight. It really suppressed his appetite and kept him awake. Everybody needs his eight hours.

Ritalin threw us for a loop. When he was about 6½ years old, he was diagnosed with ADHD, at the end of first grade. We did not involve his school. We didn't want him "labeled in any kind of public arena."

JG: *When did you notice symptoms of ADHD?*

LOLA: I always thought that there was something different about his behavior. Nobody's going to believe this,

Low DHA is Associated with ADHD

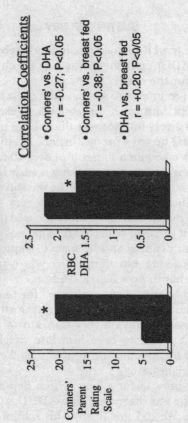

Correlation Coefficients

• Conners' vs. DHA
  r = -0.27; P<0.05

• Conners' vs. breast fed
  r = -0.38; P<0.05

• DHA vs. breast fed
  r = +0.20; P<0/05

n= 53 ADHD; 43 control

Stevens, et al. (1995) American Journal of Clinical Nutrition 62:671–678

Figure 4-1

but he was less than a year old when I thought that he behaved differently than his peers. I was told by my friends that "you're looking for problems." My son was up on his feet at a very young age, he was talking at a very young age—he's got a lot of energy. He's very quick-minded; he's very hard to keep occupied. His interest moved from thing to thing.

Other mothers will tell you that they're very proud, they're very proud that their children walked early, and talked early. They see this as a sign of intelligence. I see this as a sign of, like, my son was bored, he was dancing. He needed to find a better, faster way to explore the world. While it's not a bad thing, it's not necessarily a good thing either. Because he was never satisfied with what was in front of him. He was always looking for more. He was always looking beyond. His attention was very short.

It was hard to engage him with reading. The only thing that he would truly sit still for was TV. Television is constant motion. The slower shows he wasn't that interested in. *Sesame Street* is perfect for ADHD, since everything's in 1 or 2 minute snippets. And that's just about what he could "handle."

So, right from the beginning, I thought that there's something a little different about him. He had a very short attention span.

I started having him evaluated at a pretty young age—at 2, then at 2½. They said it was much too young, much too early to determine if there was a "real" attention problem. But . . . that couldn't really be assessed properly until school, when children are required to sit still for long periods of time, and that's when they can really start to notice who's got ADHD, and who doesn't.

JG: *And the first year of school?*

LOLA: He had a rough year, the first year. Kindergarten was very hard for him. He couldn't sit in a circle—he would push back. He couldn't sit still. He's much, much better now, but he's always been slightly off his age level. He was always behind in his age level on things like his ability to sit still, pay attention.

He's very bright; he's very articulate. He gets great marks, academically. Academically, he doesn't have a problem. Although some children have ADHD with learning disabilities, academically he's perfect. His ability to "stick with the program" has been lacking. In that regard, he's immature.

When we finally had the assessment, at age 6½, which said that he had mild-to-moderate ADHD, the doctor told us about Ritalin. We were encouraged to try Ritalin "because it really helps with these cases."

So we gave it a whirl. We kept him on it for about a week. I started him on it on a weekend. And we kept him on it for the full, following week of school. But I just couldn't bear what it was doing to him.

I will admit that there was such a big difference when he was on Ritalin. He was a different kid. He wasn't zombie-like, but he was really able to sit, and to focus, and to get his work done. I think that when he was able to screen out the distractions—that's the main problem—they're very easily distracted. He was able to learn better, and the learning had more impact, and it had more meaning.

So I was really reflective about whether we should take him off this. I mean, in the long term is Ritalin better? Will he be able to learn better on Ritalin? Maybe we can get accustomed to no appetite and his not wanting to go to sleep until midnight?

When my husband had the opportunity to spend more time with our son, he began to acknowledge that this is a real issue here. He was able to see firsthand that I wasn't "making this stuff up"—I wasn't "looking for trouble." This was a real issue, here. Our son was different.

Not bad different, he was just different. And we had to do something about this, or he *would* start to get labeled. We realized that if this went on much longer without some kind of intervention, the other kids *would* start to notice that he was different. And then it's not healthy. Then his self-esteem suffers, and all kinds of problems we don't even want to get into can come up.

JG: *So when did you find out about DHA?*

LOLA: Well, we stopped the Ritalin at about the end of first grade. Then we went through the summer "without anything." I then found out about DHA, and about the vegetable source or algae-source. So I put my son on it about a year and a half ago [as of July 1998].

So we then started second grade, and he was approaching 7. He was developmentally more mature, and was able to pay attention more. He was having fewer episodes at school that required the teacher, or school, calling. He was active, a handful, but also very gentle—he was never poking eyeballs out, and never exhibited any hyperactivity, that some children have. He's a gentle, sweet soul.

Now he's in second grade; he's showing more and more signs of maturing, I'm happy about this. And then he began to slide. His getting better was just the beginning-of-the-year resolve he had—but he could only keep it up just so long.

I'd say around Christmastime or so, going into the Christmas break, we were starting to get reports back from the teacher that he's not really sitting still, and it's becoming a bit of a distraction in class. "You know it's a huge problem," they said. He was very easily distracted, also very easily led by others. Very willing to go along, you know the "class clown," the class loved him, the kids loved him because he just makes them laugh. And that's the kinda stuff he would get in trouble for.

He was very noncompliant, not necessarily in school,

but with me. He would just dig in his heels on just about every single issue. You couldn't budge him, and it would just escalate into an argument. It was always unpleasant when he would get like this. It's pretty universal with kids that have ADHD. This is one of the hallmarks of kids with ADHD—they're less compliant than other kids.

The noncompliance is the part of ADHD that can make life, at home, really miserable. The trouble at home is that they're "hell" to live with, cause you can't transition them from dinner, to bath, to bed. Every activity, and every transition, becomes very protracted. Everything has be done in baby steps, at least at the age 5 to 7.

Everything had to be "baby steps." You can't go from dinner to the bath; you gotta go from dinner, to some quiet play, to some television, to lots of warnings, like "okay, you're going to have an hour of television" or "okay, now you've got a half hour more of television." You can't say: "You're going to have an hour of television," and then when the hour is over, say, "the hour is up, you have to take a bath, now."

Because they're not aware that an hour has gone by. Now you're asking them to transition very quickly. You have to try to help them transition every step of the way—with lots of warnings and breaks, and changing the routine as often as you can, on your way to something else. That's what made it hard at home.

The part of ADHD that makes life at school miserable is that they can't concentrate, and they start to be labeled as "dumb," they can't "keep up," which is ironic, or tragic, since, collectively, their I.Q.s are probably way above the norm. But they can't sit still and pay attention to one thing for very long. That's the trouble with ADHD at school.

So I thought: we really need to do something here. This is really not age-appropriate, and we could see that some intervention was required.

At around this time, I had been learning about DHA, and I decided to give it a try in the early spring. I'd say he probably started in March of 1997. And I saw almost instantaneous improvement. He seemed calmer.

And the one thing that I noticed almost instantaneously was an improvement in compliance. And I thought, even if it doesn't get any better than this, even if this *just* helps with the compliance issue, I will be very happy. And it also seemed to help with his ability to concentrate. And unlike Ritalin, which was, you give him the pill, and 10 minutes later, *boom,* he's doin' what he's supposed to be doin'. Very fast-acting. And a very impactful drug—it's like somebody flips a switch. At least that's what it was like for him.

JG: *Do you think of Ritalin as a form of shock treatment?*

LOLA: You know, it almost seems that way, because it really does feel like a switch is flipped. It's like, you give him the pill, and he's running around in his usual way, and like, 10 minutes later, he's kneeling on the floor, playing quietly with something that he has not looked at in 3 years.

It's like medical shock treatment. It is *that* quick. That scares me, because anything that gets to the brain, and works on the brain that quickly means, for me, that it is a very dangerous drug.

JG: *Back to DHA . . .*

LOLA: The compliance at home is what changed almost instantly with the introduction of DHA. As I said at the time: "I'll deal with the school stuff, somehow, but I can live with this."

JG: *How much did you give him?*

LOLA: I started him on 100 mg, and since he was not old enough to swallow pills at the time, I was mashing them into his applesauce every morning. He was eating it that way. Shortly thereafter, he learned to take pills on his own, and he's been taking them on his own, ever since. After he was on 100 mg for about 6 months, or so, I put him on 200 mg.

JG: *How long have you been giving him the DHA, now?*

LOLA: About a year now. You know, it's made a big difference. I have told other mothers who have children diagnosed with ADHD about DHA.

JG: *How is Justin doing today?*

LOLA: Now, he's 8½. You know what, he gets in his bed at night, and he reads! He would just never, ever, ever do this! He's a different kid. He's a fun, interesting kid, who gets in his share of trouble, which is perfectly okay with me—but it's not the wrong kind of trouble. And he's a happy kid. And I'm so *happy* that we never said anything to him like "You have ADHD." I'm so glad that he never heard those words uttered by us. Because, as it turns out, we might be able to get through his life without ever having to reveal that to him. Sometimes he asks me, "Mommy, what's so special about *these* vitamins," because I don't give him anything else. I just give him DHA. And I say "because these are the ones that are good for you, that's why."

References

Romm, Aviva Jill, *Natural Healing for Babies and Children.* Freedom, CA: The Crossing Press, 1996.

Stevens, Laura J., et al. "Essential fatty acid metabolism in boys with attention-deficit hyperactivity disorder," *American Journal of Clinical Nutrition* 62:761–768, 1995.

CHAPTER 5

·············

Vision and vision disorders: dyslexia and retinitis pigmentosa

Our sight is the most perfect and most delightful of our senses. It fills the mind with the largest variety of ideas, converses with its objects at the greatest distance, and continues the longest in action without being tired or satiated with its proper enjoyments.

Joseph Addison, *The Spectator* (c. 1711–1712)

Sight *is*, arguably, our most precious sense. It's not surprising that DHA plays a critical role in it. Let's first, though, take a quick look at vision, and how the retina and our need for DHA are intimately connected.

What is vision? It is one of the tools we use to see, navigate in, and understand the external world to the extent we can survive in a world full of natural dangers—in the shape of other living things and the environment itself.

The Retina

The components of the eye allow photons from the visual field to be projected as an image on the retina, which is around the size of a postage stamp and serves as a "movie screen" for projected images. Although the retinal surface is covered with nerve cells and blood vessels, the brain filters them out of what we see.

Photoreceptors (rods and cones) are located at the back of the retina; these are the only cells which can detect light. Intererestingly enough, the retina's photoreceptor layer contains about 120 million rods and 6 million cones, arranged side-by-side.

Photoreceptors take incoming photons and turn them into neurochemical messages. Rod photoreceptors are mostly used in low light conditions (not for color), and are very sensitive to light. The three types of cone cells—one for red light, one for green, and one for blue—are sensitive to different wavelengths, allowing us to make out colors.

In any case, signals are communicated from these photoreceptors, through what are called bipolar cells, to the ganglion (nerve) cells. These ganglion cells, which bundle together to form the optic nerve, in turn, communicate these image signals to the brain. The occipital lobes at the back of the brain process all of the pieces of information (signals) it receives through the optic nerve. The result: an image!

Enter DHA

The retina's photoreceptor outer segment membranes contain one of the body's highest concentrations of DHA (over 50 percent) in the body. It's no surprise then that studies on retinal function—and vision—have also looked at omega–3 levels, particularly supplemental DHA.

In nonhuman primates deficient in dietary omega–3 fats, for example, there are "profound biochemical changes in the fatty-acid composition of the membranes of the retina." These changes are demonstrated by three symptoms: visual impairment, poor electroretinogram results (measuring retinal function by flashing a light), and—strangely—polydipsia (excessive thirst), as William E. Connor, M.D., and colleagues, explained in a 1992 study which appeared in *Nutrition Reviews*.

In another recent animal study done in 1998, Danish researchers M. Christensen and others showed that mammals jealously hold on to high levels of DHA in the retina as long as possible. In fact, a 1998 study out of the National University of Argentina, by A. Terrasa and associates, even demonstrated that specific proteins present in the retina may act as "antioxidants," fending off free-radical-caused damage to rod outer segment membranes (Figure 5–1) for as long as they can.

How does dyslexia fit in?

One theory holds that people with dyslexia may be less able to process visual information than are nondyslexics, particularly that information which allows us to adapt to dark conditions.

With 10 percent of the U.S. population suffering from dyslexia (and 4 percent severely affected), it appears that this problem is becomng more common.

"In the U.S., there has been a three-fold increase in the prevalence of dyslexia—the number of new cases in the community, between 1976 and 1993," said B. Jacqueline Stordy, Ph.D., who's based in England.

Fortunately, DHA supplements may improve the "central deficit" in the processing system that may be behind dyslexia.

In the August 5, 1995, edition of the prestigious mainstream British medical journal, *The Lancet*, in fact, Stordy reported on her research using DHA supplementation in adults with dyslexia.

For one month, five patients with dyslexia were given 480 mg of DHA every day (five people with dyslexia—the controls—were not). In the dyslexic patients given DHA, dark-adaptation ability (scotopic vision) was "consistently and significantly improved."

Role of DHA in the ROS of the Retina

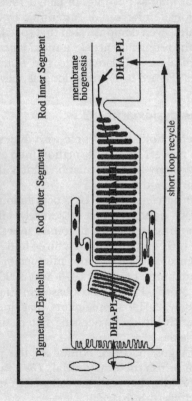

Pigmented Epithelium   Rod Outer Segment   Rod Inner Segment

membrane biogenesis

DHA-PL

DHA-PL

short loop recycle

After Bazan (1989)

Figure 5-1

Stordy also has found that "DHA supplements given to dyslexics can also be associated with improvements in reading ability and behavior." Some of these findings await further confirmation by formal, controlled studies, although they are clearly very promising.

Retinitis Pigmentosa

Another interesting area of DHA/vision research includes studies which have looked at fatty acid and DHA levels in patients with a condition called **retinitis pigmentosa** (RP), a hereditary degenerative disease of the retina which brings on such problems as: night blindness, pigmentation changes in the retina, narrowing of the field of vision, and loss of vision. These conditions stem from the breakdown of photoreceptors.

In a July 27, 1998, conversation, Dennis Hoffman, Ph.D., of the Retina Foundation of the Southwest, described the progression of RP this way: Night blindness is typically the first symptom, which comes about as rods (responsible for contrast vision) on the periphery of the retina "die." As this occurs, surrounding cone receptors also atrophy. The loss of cone cells in the peripheral retina leads to tunnel vision, as these cells control our acute and color vision. As the tunnel vision gets worse, legal blindness, and often total blindness, follow.

Although "the cause" of RP is blamed on specific genetic mutations, factors such as the environment, metabolism, and diet apparently determine the *severity* of the disease in those who have it.

Within the factor of diet, the fatty acid status of membranes in the photoreceptor influence how well the retina functions.

The research

In 1992, Junxian Gong and associates, of the Tufts University School of Medicine, looked at 188 patients with various forms of retinitis pigmentosa and 91 patients without RP in regard to DHA levels.

The authors found that patients with a strong genetically caused form of RP (X-linked) had DHA levels in plasma "that were significantly lower than normal."

In 1995, Ernst J. Schaefer and others looked at levels of DHA in phosphatidylethanolamine (PE) within red blood cells (RBC), because PE is "abundant" in cell membranes, and is "markedly enriched in DHA, especially within rod outer segment membranes in the retina."

They studied 155 patients with retinitis and 101 patients without RP. They found that DHA levels were decreased across-the-board in the subjects with retinitis. Based on their results, the authors suggest that these fatty acid "abnormalities" may actually contribute to the progression of this condition.

In that same year (1995), Dennis Hoffman and University of Texas medical researcher David Birch also examined DHA levels in red blood cells. In fact, they looked at 18 patients with X-linked retinitis and 28 patients without RP.

These authors confirmed that the "overwhelming majority" of patients with retinitis have lower levels of DHA compared to normally sighted control patients. Hoffman and Birch suggested, at that time, that a "defect" in fatty acid chain metabolism is probably behind the problem.

DHA supplementation

What was groundbreaking about the conclusions Hoffman and Birch drew was their call for DHA supplementation. As they put it: "Dietary supplementation of DHA [. . .] may restore blood levels of DHA to normal, regardless of the specific mechanism impaired in the disease."

And then they added this: "It now becomes important to consider the potential for early nutritional intervention to delay" the degenerative rod loss in patients with X-linked RP.

Nevertheless, in terms of actual results from DHA supplementation, the jury's not in quite yet, according to Hoffman and Birch. Now while they *are* supplementing patients with DHA—with funding from the Foundation Fighting Blindness and the Orphan Products Division of the U.S. Food and Drug Administration (FDA)—the results of the study won't be available until the year 2000.

Meanwhile, the possibilities remain very exciting.

References

Christensen, M.M., et al. "Dietary structured triacylglycerols containing docosahexaenoic acid given from birth affect visual and auditory performance and tissue fatty acid profiles of rats," *Journal of Nutrition* 128(6): 1011–1017, June 1998.

Connor, William E., M.D., et al. "Essential fatty acids: the importance of omega–3 fatty acids in the retina and brain," *Nutrition Reviews* 50(4):21–29, 1992.

Gong, Junxian, et al. "Plasma docosahexaenoic acid levels in various genetic forms of retinitis pigmentosa," *Investigative Ophthalmology & Visual Science* 33(9):2596–2602, 1992.

Hoffman, Dennis R., Ph.D., and Birch, David G. "Docosahexaenoic acid in red blood cells of patients with X-linked retinitis pigmentosa," *Investigative Ophthalmology & Visual Science* 36(6):1009–1018, 1995.

Schaefer, Ernst J., et al. "Red blood cell membrane phosphatidylethanolamine fatty acid content in various forms of retinitis pigmentosa," *Journal of Lipid Research* 36:1427–1433, 1995.

Terrasa, A., et al. "Lipoperoxidation of rod outer segments of bovine retina is inhibited by soluble binding proteins for fatty acids," *Mol Cell Biochem* 178(1-2):181–186, January 1998.

PART III

▼

Metabolic and Peroxisomal Disorders

DHA's influence on the body is far-reaching and profound. What our bodies are able to accomplish with fatty acids becomes all the more apparent when we see the tragic, sometimes fatal, consequences that result from conditions in which our bodies cannot properly make use of these fats—in cases of what, in medicalese, are called: in-born "errors" of metabolism and peroxisome-assembly defects.

First off, let's refresh ourselves as to what metabolism and peroxisomes are. **Metabolism** really encompasses all biochemical reactions in the body, especially as they relate to the interface of nutrition and energy. Metabolism consists of *anabolism*, an energy-draining process which involves building small molecules into larger structures (like amino acids into proteins), and *catabolism*, an energy-producing process which involves breaking down large structures into small molecules (like glycogen down to pyruvic acid). There are many subtypes of metabolism, including: carbohydrate, electrolyte, fat, protein, and respiratory. **Peroxisomes** are subcellular units, or organelles, which perform a multitude of essential metabolic reactions.

We'll be looking at DHA and rather rare (yet very serious) diseases that involve problems in fat-metabolism and "peroxisome assembly," problems which often lead to fatal diseases in early childhood, including:

- Long-Chain 3–Hydroxyacyl-CoA Dehydrogenase Deficiency (LCHADD);
- Adrenoleukodystrophy (ALD);
- Zellweger/Pseudo-Zellweger Syndromes and Juvenile Neuronal Ceroid Lipofuscinosis (JNCL) or Batten's Disease; and
- Phenylketonuria (PKU) or Phenylpyruvic Oligophrenia.

CHAPTER 6

....

LCHADD

*We were hoping to make a difference, but we were not
expecting this. The great thing is that we're going
to really help these kids, and it looks as if we're going
to learn more about DHA metabolism in the
process.*

Melanie Gillingham, Ph.D. Cand., July 30, 1998

Long-chain 3–hydroxyacyl-CoA dehydrogenase deficiency (LCHADD) is a big name for a serious disease
which primarily afflicts some of the smallest members
of our population, mostly babies and children under 3
years of age. LCHADD is a very rare, inherited metabolic
disorder marked by the body's complete lack of a mitochondrial enzyme which serves as its namesake. This
enzyme is needed to break down fats for energy; that's
why this disorder is also referred to as a fatty acid oxidation disorder.

There are about 75 diagnosed cases of LCHADD
in the United States (and about 200 in Europe). The
symptoms usually present themselves in infancy or early
childhood. Major symptoms include (but are not limited
to): hypoketotic hypoglycemia, early-onset cardiomyopathy (heart condition due to enlargement of the muscles
of the heart), hepatic (liver) dysfunction, peripheral
neuropathy (nerve problems, possibly due to demyelination), infections of the upper respiratory tract and
gastrointestinal tract, hypotonia (muscle weakness), and
retinal degeneration. In the first few weeks of life,
infants with this disorder may "feed poorly, vomit fre-

quently and not gain" enough weight, according to the National Organization for Rare Disorders.

In terms of LCHADD, one of the first researchers to stumble onto the benefits of supervised supplementation with DHA was Ingrid Tein, M.D., of Toronto's Hospital for Sick Children. Tein "instituted a trial of docosahexaenoic acid [DHA] therapy, which has resulted in a clinical improvement in the peripheral neuropathy," suggesting measured supplementation with DHA.

Research News

On July 30, 1998, I had a conversation with Melanie Gillingham, a doctoral student in nutrition at the University of Wisconsin's Biochemical Genetics Program (Waisman Center), who works with LCHADD.

JG: *How did you get into this LCHADD research?*

Gillingham: Well, I was doing a fellowship at the Waisman Center, which is a center for children with different developmental diseases. Since I was trained as a nutritionist, I was counseling some patients in the clinic who have LCHADD.

JG: *How did DHA enter the picture?*

Gillingham: We had the LCHADD children on very low-fat diets, since they can't oxidize fat. Concerned that the children, very conceivably, might become deficient in essential fatty acids, we measured their plasma essential fatty acids and saw that their DHA levels were very low.

JG: *What then?*

Gillingham: First off, we did various diet manipulations and, no matter what we did to the diets, the DHA levels never came up.

Well, I visited our medical library and began to pore over the DHA research, with a particular focus on the vision studies, since one of the long-term complications of LCHADD is retinal degeneration, a problem which can eventually lead to blindness. At that point, nobody really knew what the relation between the vision problems and the fat-enzyme defect was.

So, over a two-year period, we tried to get a patient's DHA levels up with diet, but couldn't do it. We then thought that there must be some specific relation between this enzyme defect and the patient's inability to make DHA the way most of us should be able to.

JG: *Was this when your study began?*

Gillingham: Yes. We actually started an open-label trial with no control, since we wanted all of the patients to benefit, if there was to be a benefit. As of today, we have 10 children from all across the country who are enrolled in our study. We use 60–120 mg of DHA oil, depending on body weight.

They come to Wisconsin, and we baseline test them before they start DHA. We measure their visual evoked potential, their electroretinograms, and use a whole battery of eye exams. We then see them at the Waisman Center, where we evaluate their LCHADD status.

The children come back at 6 months, and then we repeat the whole series, and then again at the one-year mark. After that, they come back yearly.

JG: *Are you seeing improvement?*

Gillingham: Well, right now, we have three children who've been on DHA for 2 years. In all three cases, their eyes (that is, via the results of their electroretinograms) have significantly improved—far more than the electrophysiologist had ever expected. So their visual acuity has significantly improved.

We've also seen some real dramatic improvement in "visual evoked potential." We test visual evoked potential with an electroencephalogram and by stimulation of the retina with a light flashing at quarter-second intervals. A normal visual evoked potential is around 30. Our kids were starting at numbers like 9, 15, and 20. All of them are now close to 30 (Figure 6–1).

I also have four other children who've been on DHA for about 6 months at this point. Of those four children, three have improved in the same way as in our first group.

JG: *This must be very exciting for you!*

Gillingham: I'm thrilled! We were hoping to make a difference, but we were definitely not expecting *this!* The great thing is that we're going to really help these kids, and it looks as if we're going to learn more about DHA metabolism in the process.

We're also going to be looking at whether this intervention with DHA needs to be done when these children are very young, or if benefits can be achieved when they're older.

References

Gillingham, M.B., et al. "DHA supplementation in children with long-chain 3–hydroxyacyl-CoA dehydrogenase deficiency." Presented at the seventh International Congress of Inborn Errors of Metabolism, May 21–25, 1997, Vienna, Austria.

Tein, Ingrid, M.D. "Clinical, enzymatic and treatment aspects of long-chain L-3–hydroxyacyl-CoA dehydrogenase deficiency." [Abstract, no other data available]

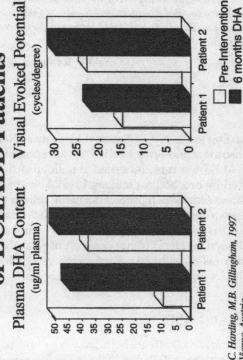

DHA Supplementation of LCHADD Patients

Plasma DHA Content
(ug/ml plasma)

Visual Evoked Potential
(cycles/degree)

☐ Pre-Intervention
■ 6 months DHA

C. Harding, M.B. Gillingham, 1997
Vienna, Austria

Figure 6-1

CHAPTER 7

....

ALD

There's been a literal explosion in understanding the genetic basis of peroxisomal disorders, but the use of these polyunsaturated fatty acids, specifically DHA, is one of the few therapeutic avenues that has gotten anybody excited.

Gerald V. Raymond, M.D., 1998

According to the NIH's National Institute of Neurological Disorders and Stroke (NINDS), adrenoleukodystrophy (ALD) is a rare, inherited genetic disorder that is marked by two bodily changes: breakdown of the fatty myelin sheaths which protect the nerve cells in the brain and progressive malfunctioning of the adrenal gland.

ALD is one of a group of genetic disorders called **"leukodystrophies,"** which cause damage to the myelin sheaths (as mentioned), fatty coverings which serve as insulators for the nerve fibers in the brain.

Neonatal ALD

Neonatal ALD affects both baby boys and baby girls, with symptoms which can include the following: "mental retardation, facial abnormalities, seizures, retinal degeneration, hypotonia (low muscle tone), hepatomegaly (enlarged liver), and adrenal" malfunctioning, as the NINDS explains.

Childhood ALD

Childhood ALD is the most severe form of the disorder. It affects only boys, usually beginning between the ages of 4 and 10 years. Features of this form of the disorder may include: visual loss, learning disabilities, seizures, poorly articulated speech, difficulty swallowing, deafness, disturbances of gait and coordination, fatigue, intermittent vomiting, increased skin pigmentation, and progressive dementia. There is an *adult-onset* form of ALD as well, usually beginning between ages 21 and 35.

According to Hugo W. Moser, M.D., of Baltimore's Kennedy-Krieger Institute, X-linked adrenoleukodystrophy (X-ALD) is the most common peroxisomal disorder, and is characterized by the accumulation of saturated very-long-chain fatty acids, specifically hexacosanoic acid (a 26–carbon fat) and tetracosanoic acid (a 24–carbon fat) due to a problem forming a derivative of these fatty acids in the peroxisome.

In about 50 percent of the patients, these super-long-chain fats often bring on an inflammatory/immune response similar to that seen in multiple sclerosis and is associated with rapid neurological breakdown.

Treatment?

One approach is to give a special mixture of glyceryl trioleate and glyceryl trierucate oils, also known as Lorenzo's Oil, combined with dietary restriction of saturated VLCFAs.

Many of us remember George Miller's powerful 1993 movie, *Lorenzo's Oil*, which told the story of Lorenzo Odone (played by Zack O'Malley Greenburg), a boy who was diagnosed, in 1985, with ALD, and the desperate struggle of his parents Augusto and Michaela Odone (played by Nick Nolte and Susan Sarandon) to find some way to save him—Lorenzo's Oil is what they discovered.

Nevertheless, Moser tells us that, while this Lorenzo's Oil therapy normalizes the levels of saturated VLCFAs in plasma, "recent data indicate that the oil does not enter the brain," and, apparently, is not able to significantly improve the clinical progression of the disease in patients who already are experiencing nerve degeneration. On the other hand, if therapy is begun before neurological symptoms start, the frequency of episodes and more general severity of neurological disability can be reduced. Bone marrow transplantation has helped some carefully selected patients in reducing the frequency of episodes and severity of neurological disability as well.

Could DHA be the missing piece of the puzzle? Enter Manuela Martinez, M.D., and Gerald Raymond, M.D.

A breakthrough occurs

In 1993, Dr. Martinez, of Barcelona's Hospital de Tarrasa, and colleagues published a landmark study in the journal, *Neurology,* outlining their successful results with one patient with neonatal ALD.

According to Martinez, patients in the neonatal group "seem to have a defect in peroxisomal" assembly, the exact cause of which is unknown. She also explained that these patients have a "profound deficiency of [DHA]."

"Since DHA is considered to be a very important constituent of nerves and retinal cell membranes," Martinez said, "such a deficiency could, at least, in part, explain the mental retardation and visual defects in these patients, and may even play a role in their abnormal peroxisomal" assembly.

In fact, with one 6-year-old boy, Martinez did the following. She gave to the child a pure DHA preparation, going from 50 mg/day to 250 mg/day. After only 6 weeks of treatment, Martinez found some of the DHA levels and fat ratios, had balanced out. After one year of DHA treatment, the boy is remarkably improved: He has much less spasticity (especially in the upper limbs); he can handle, and manipulate, small objects; he can drink without help; and his vision has improved (as measured by "visual evoked potentials").

Having seen slides of this little boy before and after treatment with DHA, I can say that the improvement was dramatic.

The authors concluded that: "These results raise new hopes about the treatment of peroxisomal disorders."

Research News

On July 31, 1998, I had a conversation with Dr. Gerald Raymond, of the Kennedy-Krieger Institute, about his current work in the area of children with ALD.

JG: *What got you into ALD research?*

Raymond: We were looking at the work of Dr. Manuela Martinez, who showed that children who do not make peroxisomes, or children who have peroxisome-assembly defects, do not make adequate amounts of DHA, and, in fact, have low levels of all of the polyunsaturated fatty acids in brain tissue, liver, and other tissues of the body.

Meanwhile, through some complicated biochemistry, others were able to show that the "last stages" of DHA are actually produced in the peroxisome. We already know that it's through the process of beta-oxidation, or breaking down of a longer-chain fatty acid, that DHA is formed.

Now Martinez supplemented people with these disorders. Remember that children with peroxisome-assembly disorders, such as Zellweger's syndrome, are profoundly retarded, have retinitis pigmentosa, and other retinal abnormalities. Although there are milder cases, all have some degree of visual and mental handicap.

Since Martinez was successful in bringing up DHA levels, it became apparent that supplementing these patients would be worthwhile. She achieved success in several patients, results on two of whom she published. Although she said that she believes that DHA-supplementation is a "successful therapy," there are others who have been more skeptical.

JG: *And you?*

Raymond: We chose two tacks, one of which involved trying to reproduce some of this work, including an open-dosing study which we did over the last couple of years.

JG: *What did you find?*

Raymond: We were able to show that we could raise DHA and arachidonic acid levels.

While we can raise serum levels, we can't know, of course, how well we're raising levels in the brain and retina. So we're presently running a placebo-controlled, blinded study in children with peroxisome-assembly disorders, looking at retinal function and neuro-developmental function.

We do our double-blinded study over a one-year period of time. At the end of the year, the children are placed on DHA until the completion of the study. We also carry out electrophysiologic and developmental studies on the eye.

That's how we got into DHA and peroxisomal disorders, and that's precisely where our work is focusing.

JG: *I know that you're awaiting the results of your study, but how do you see the value of therapeutic DHA supplementation in babies, and children, with peroxisome-assembly problems?*

Raymond: Well, I must admit that DHA supplementation is one of the few promising therapies for peroxisomal disorders at this moment. There's been a literal explosion in understanding the genetic basis of peroxisomal disorders, but the use of these polyunsaturated fatty acids, specifically DHA, is one of the few therapeutic avenues that has gotten anybody excited.

References

Ebert, Roger. *Lorenzo's Oil* [movie review], *Chicago Sun-Times,* January 15, 1993.

Martinez, Manuela, M.D., et al. "Docosahexaenoic acid—a new therapeutic approach to peroxisomal-disorder patients: experience with two cases," *Neurology* 43:1389–1397, 1993.

National Institute of Neurological Disorders and Stroke (NINDS). "Adrenoleukodystrophy." Bethesda, MD: National Institutes of Health (NIH), September 1997. Website: *http://www.ninds.nih.gov/HEALINFO/DISORDER/Adrenoleukodystrophy/adrenoleuko.htm.*

Raymond, Gerald, M.D., et al. "Docosahexaenoic acid therapy in peroxisome biogenesis disorders." [No other data available]

CHAPTER 8

Zellweger/Pseudo-Zellweger syndromes and JNCL/Batten's disease

While waiting for some light to clarify this fascinating issue, it seems worthwhile testing the possible beneficial effects of a diet rich in docosahexaenoic acid in peroxisomal patients.

Manuela Martinez, M.D., 1991

Zellweger Syndromes

Zellweger syndrome is a rare, congenital disorder characterized by a reduced level, or absence, of peroxisomes. Zellweger syndrome is another of the "leukodystrophies" that break down the myelin sheath covering nerves in the brain.

The most common features of this syndrome include an enlarged liver, high levels of iron and copper in the blood, and vision disturbances. Other symptoms may include the following: unusual facial characteristics, mental retardation, seizures, an inability to suck and/or swallow, lack of muscle tone (and inability to move), jaundice, gastrointestinal bleeding, and lack of prenatal growth. Death typically occurs by 6 months after the beginning of symptoms.

In Zellweger syndrome, liver peroxisomes are virtually absent, and some lipid enzymes are deficient; as a result, there is a tissue accumulation of very-long-chain fatty acids and a decrease in plasmalogen levels (plasmalogens being special phospholipids in which a fatty acid group is replaced by reactive organic compounds

produced by the breakdown of alcohols, called alde-
hydes).

In **Pseudo-Zellweger syndrome,** on the other hand,
peroxisomes are present, although the clinical picture
is similar to those with classic Zellweger syndrome. This
variation of Zellweger syndrome appears to involve an
isolated deficiency of one peroxisome enzyme (peroxisomal 3–oxoacyl-CoA thiolase), a buildup of a couple
of the very-long-chain fats, and, unexpectedly, normal
plasmalogen levels.

In 1991, a study by Manuela Martinez, M.D. (whose
ALD work we discussed earlier in Chapter 7), looked
at 34 infants, from 26 prenatal weeks to 2 years of age,
in addition to 3 cases in the age range of 4–8 years.

In four patients with peroxisomal disorders, Martinez demonstrated important PUFA abnormalities,
"mainly consisting of a drastic decrease in the tissue
levels of [DHA]."

In Martinez' study as well, specifically in three
patients with Zellweger syndrome and one with Pseudo-
Zellweger syndrome, she again found "the most significant abnormality as a sizable decrease in the brain levels
of [DHA]."

Her analysis of the patients led to this convincing
statement: "[. . .] given the importance of [DHA] in
[brain] and [retinal] membranes, the deficiency of
[DHA] could explain much of the neurological and
visual symptoms in peroxisomal patients." She went on
to add that "even the myelination" problems could, at
least partly, "be explained by a [DHA] deficiency, since
the [fatty acid] content of [. . .] myelin seems to be
particularly affected in omega–3 deprivation."

Martinez concluded that: "The existence of such
profound alterations in the PUFA composition of tissues
opens new avenues for research in the field of peroxisomal disorders." And: "While waiting for some light
to clarify this fascinating issue, it seems worthwhile test-

ing the possible beneficial effects of a diet rich in [DHA]" in patients with peroxisome disorders.

JNCL/Batten's Disease

Our preliminary evidence in this small group of patients suggests that therapy with PUFAs may have slowed down the disease process, and even halted it in the younger patients

Michael J. Bennett, et al., 1994

Juvenile Neuronal Ceroid Lipofuscinosis, also called **Batten's disease,** is another of the group of severe, inherited neuro-degenerative diseases for which the underlying cause is unknown.

According to the National Organization for Rare Disorders, the disease, in whatever type, is marked by accumulation of a fatty substance (lipopigment) in the brain and non-nerve-containing tissue. This disorder in storing lipopigment is characterized by rapidly progressive vision failure (optic atrophy) and neurological problems.

Occurring mainly in families of Northern European (Scandinavian) ancestry, Batten's disease may also cause deterioration of normal intellect functioning along with the neurological problems typical of the disease.

Usually, patients begin in early childhood (mostly before 8 years of age) with retinal degeneration, and, according to Michael J. Bennett's 1994 study, then suffer "gradual destruction of rods and cones leading to blindness." This is followed by seizures and other neurological disturbances, culminating in spastic paralysis of all limbs, and death, in the second or third decade of life.

In 1993, A. Kohlschütter and associates of the University of Hamburg, Germany, measured phospholipid and lipid levels in 11 patients with Batten's disease, aged 9 to 24 years, and in control patients who were either healthy or with other disorders.

In addition to low levels of various phospholipids, levels of DHA (and total levels of omega–3s) were found to be "abnormally low" in patients with Batten's disease, whether they were being treated with anticonvulsant drugs or not. Since linoleic acid (parent omega–6) was normal in all groups, omega–6 deficiency is clearly not an issue.

Supplementation begins

In the following year, 1994, Michael J. Bennett and colleagues took the 1993 findings to the next level—actually supplementing these patients with omega–3 polyunsaturated fats (PUFAs). They found some startling results.

"Since polyunsaturated fatty acids (PUFAs) are the fatty acids of greatest importance to many membrane functions [. . .], we attempted to modify these membrane abnormalities by dietary PUFA supplementation," the authors explained.

The results were so positive that the authors concluded their study in this manner. "Our preliminary evidence in this small group of patients suggests that therapy with [omega–3] PUFAs may have slowed down the disease process, and even halted it in the younger patients."

The authors can't understand why other hospitals, research centers, and physicians don't try omega–3 PUFA supplementation in patients with neonatal and juvenile Batten's disease, since it's "rational, inexpensive, and harmless."

References

Bennett, M.J., et al. "Juvenile neuronal ceroid-lipofuscinosis: developmental progress after supplementation with polyunsaturated fatty acids," *Developmental Medical Child Neurology* 36(7):630–638, 1994.

Kohlschütter, A., et al. "Low erythrocyte plasmalogen and plasma docosahexaenoic acid (DHA) in Juvenile Neuronal Ceroid-lipofuscinosis (JNCL)," *Journal of Inherited Metabolic Disorders* 16:299–304, 1993.

Martinez, Manuela, M.D., et al. "Developmental profiles of polyunsaturated fatty acids in the brain of normal infants and patients with peroxisomal diseases: severe deficiency of docosahexaenoic acid in Zellweger's and Pseudo-Zellweger's syndromes." In: Simopoulos, A.P., et al. (editors): *Health Effects of Omega–3 Polyunsaturated Fatty Acids in Seafoods. Volume 66: World Review of Nutrition and Dietetics.* Basel, Switzerland: S. Karger, 1991.

CHAPTER 9

······································

PKU/Folling's disease

Since docosahexaenoic and arachidonic acids are fundamental structural components for normal brain development, it seems necessary to consider a dietary adjustment in these patients.

P. Sanjurjo, et al., 1994

PKU, also called **Folling's disease** and phenylpyruvic oligophrenia, stands for: phenylketonuria. PKU is an inherited inability to break down the amino acid, phenylalanine. In normal function, phenylalanine is broken down into tyrosine, another amino acid, by a specific amino acid enzyme—phenylalanine hydroxylase.

Unfortunately, this enzyme is inactive in people with PKU. Because of this metabolic monkey wrench, or block, extremely high levels of phenylalanine build up in the blood plasma, spinal fluid, and urine.

In the body's tissues, the excess amino acid, and its abnormal breakdown products (metabolites), interfere with different metabolic tasks. The central nervous system is affected, too: mental retardation, epileptic seizures, and abnormal brain-wave patterns can result.

Symptoms

Generally, the first physical signs of nerve cell damage are seen in young infants 4 to 6 months old. The excess storage of high levels of phenylalanine in body tissues often leads to a decrease in the formation of one product of tyrosine, melanin, the pigment found in the skin, hair, and eyes. This is said to explain why people with PKU normally have blond hair, blue eyes, and fair skin.

The majority of cases of PKU are discovered in the newborn period, before clinical symptoms appear. In any case, it's estimated that one in 10,000 newborns have excessively high plasma phenylalanine levels; out of these, about 66 percent will have the classic form of PKU, which, if untreated, will cause severe mental retardation.

Treatment?

Traditionally, a diet low in phenylalanine is effective in controlling the body's level of this amino acid. Such a diet, which should be continued until adolescence, typically calls for quite stringent measures, including: no meat, no dairy, no high-protein foods. In terms of protein needs, doctors commonly prescribe a phenylalanine-free protein drink.

Pregnant women who have PKU are also advised to *restart* this diet (before conception, at best, and no later than the first weeks of the first trimester) in order to control their own abnormally high levels of phenylalanine, which can severely harm an unborn child, leading to their baby being born with one or another abnormality, including: microcephaly (abnormally small head), mental retardation, congenital heart disease, and intrauterine growth retardation. Other, associated problems can include: abnormal gait, stance, and sitting posture; eczema; and epilepsy. Further associations with cataracts and brain calcification haven't been conclusively proven or disproven as yet.

First discovered in Norway, a disproportionally large percentage of PKU carriers also appear to have lineage traceable to Celtic origins, specifically from Ireland and western Scotland.

Modern research and fatty acids

In 1994, P. Sanjurjo, et al., from the Hospital de Cruces (Baracaldo) of the Basque University School of Medicine (Bilbao), both in Spain's province of Vizcaya, carried out an important study on 40 patients with PKU.

The study group was made up of 15 female and 25 male patients, who ranged in age from 2 months to 20 years, although only five of the people were over 14 years of age; the control group consisted of 50 children without PKU.

The analysis the researchers conducted showed that the children with PKU had higher than normal levels of the omega–6 fat, linoleic acid, and much lower than normal levels of DHA, compared to the control group. The PKU patients also tended to have lower levels of DHA's parent fat, eicosapentaenoic acid (EPA). In terms of red cell membrane levels of fats, the PKU children also had heightened levels of the omega–6 arachidonic acid.

The authors showed that the relatively high intake of the omega–6 linoleic acid "causes a major imbalance in the [fatty acid] profile of PKU patients" that immediately results in too much linoleic acid in plasma, a serious deficiency of DHA, and, to a lesser extent, a lowered level of arachidonic acid.

Sanjurjo and his colleagues concluded their research with this finding: "Since docosahexaenoic and arachidonic acids are fundamental structural components for normal brain development, it seems necessary to consider a dietary adjustment in these patients," such a dietary adjustment consisting of: (1) supplementation with pure DHA, and (2) reduction of omega–6 fats, especially linoleic acid.

Good news with maternal omega–3 supplementation!

In the same year Sanjurjo's article appeared, M. Giovannini and others from Italy's University of Milan reported a fascinating case of successful omega–3/DHA intervention in a woman with PKU.

They report the case of a 29-year-old woman, who had been diagnosed with classic PKU at 9 months of age (since she then had plasma phenylalanine levels of 1200 micromoles per liter). A low-phenylalanine diet was soon introduced, which allowed her to achieve good metabolic control and normal neurological/psychomotor development.

Unfortunately, when she reached the age of 9 years, her parents stopped her special diet, against the advice of the authors (her physicians). When she was 27, she married a healthy male and, fortunately, returned to the authors' care. With the active care of her physicians, she planned her pregnancy in such a way that she could have a full 12 months of the low-phenylalanine diet before conception. Her plasma-phenylalanine levels dropped to 120 mmol/L, a normal level, and remained stable throughout her baby's gestation.

From about the fifth month of pregnancy, a special grouping of omega–3 fats was also added to her daily diet, which included: 240 mg of DHA's "grandma" fat, alpha-linolenic acid; 360 mg of DHA's parent, EPA; and 240 mg of DHA, in addition to a small quantity of the 18-carbon fat, stearidonic acid. She continued this supplementation until delivery.

The results? Beautiful! Her little boy was born 100

percent normal, in all respects: weight, length, measurements, and later mental/neurological development.

Hopefully, a result like this will change the world's dietary protocol for prospective mothers with PKU. The result was nothing short of miraculous.

References

Giovannini, M., et al. "Fatty acid supplementation in a case of maternal phenylketonuria," [short report] *Journal of Inherited Metabolic Disorders* 17:630–631, 1994.

Sanjurjo, P., Perteagudo, L., Rodríguez Soriano, J., Vilaseca, A., and Campistol, J. "Polyunsaturated fatty acid status in patients with phenylketonuria," *Journal of Inherited Metabolic Disorders* 17:704–709, 1994.

PART IV

▼

Immunity, Inflammation and Cardiovascular Health

Okay, so you're asking: What do these things have in common? Plenty. In fact, there are few examples where the incredible connectivity, overlapping and intersecting of all of our health (homeostasis or balance) and unhealth (disease or imbalance) vectors is more apparent than in the interface between immune/allergic response, inflammation, and cardiovascular function.

In Chapter 10, we'll review the wide array of diseases and disorders, of immunity, inflammation, and allergy. It's the inclusion of Chapter 11—Cardiovascular Health—in this section which may be a shocker to some, but it shouldn't be, since some of the same components which signal, mediate, and modulate immune, inflammatory, and allergic responses also signal, mediate and modulate circulation and vascular response.

We see a number of the same players in all of these activities: eicosanoids (like the prostaglandins and thromboxane) and cytokines (like interleukin–1 [Il–1], and tumor necrosis factor, TNF). In recent years, it has become increasingly clear that polyunsaturated fatty acids are key in both producing these mediators (prostaglandins)—which, in turn, influence immune function (like T-cells)—and in modulating inflammatory/immune response (suppressing or stimulating those cytokines, for example). In fact, the eicosanoids regulate many cell functions and play critical roles in wide-ranging activities, including various immune and inflammatory functions.

When we realize that IL–1 and TNF contribute to both the "pathogenesis of inflammatory disease" and atherosclerosis, we see clearly how intimately intertwined are immunity, inflammation, allergy, and cardiovascular function—and how dietary supplementation with DHA can help keep them, and us, healthy!

CHAPTER 10

....

Diseases of immunity, inflammation, and allergy

Our immune strength is directly influenced by certain choices we make.
By choosing to protect and nourish our immune system, we can harness the body's innate power to heal.

Kenneth Bock, M.D., and Nellie Sabin,
The Road to Immunity, 1997

Many studies have shown that supplementation with fish oil or DHA reduces acute and chronic inflammation and rebalances our immune response. Nutritionist P.C. Calder, for example, of the University of Southampton, U.K., noted this in a 1997 article "Omega–3 polyunsaturated fatty acids and cytokine production in health and disease."

The eosinophil connection? The overaccumulation of immune factors, called eosinophils, has been linked to the development of allergic diseases, according to S. Kikuchi, et al., from the Nagoya University School of Medicine, Japan, in a study published in March 1998.

In this animal study, DHA administration decreased hyperimmune/hyperallergic response "big time," depending on how much was given. These authors concluded their research in this fashion: "Our results suggest a possible mechanism for the improvement of allergic diseases by dietary supplementation with [omega–3] PUFAs."

Cancer

Breast cancer

As noted Japanese researcher, M. Noguchi, said in 1995, the medical literature has pretty well established that omega–3 PUFAs, primarily DHA, hold down (or suppress) breast cancer development in general and the spread of tumor cells in particular. More recent research by an American counterpart—N. Simonsen, of the University of North Carolina, in 1998—has even proposed that the actual omega–6 to omega–3 ratio in breast adipose tissue itself is involved in providing an inhospitable environment for tumors to start, grow, and spread (if the omega–3 ratio is high enough).

Colon cancer metastasis

A fascinating study from 1997, by M. Iigo and colleagues, of the National Cancer Center in Japan, demonstrated that DHA showed "marked" antimetastatic [antitumor spread] activity against colon carcinoma 26. This very interesting result is probably due to the way in which DHA transforms the tumor cell membrane so that the tumor cell then has a "decreased ability to metastasize."

Iigo's conclusion is backed up by even more recent research out of Japan. From the department of surgery, University of Tokyo, W.S. Tsai and associates have shown that DHA "appears to have specific [blocking] effects on cancer cells and may, thus, enhance the host defense against colon cancer."

Liver cancer

In a 1998 study out of Rome, EPA and DHA were found to discourage cancer cell growth (proliferation), but in different ways. While EPA seems to block cell proliferation, DHA appears to encourage cancer cells to meet an early demise (through something called "apoptosis").

Generalized malignancy

A 1998 study out of the University Medical School, Patras, Greece, by C.A. Gogos and colleagues, focused on 60 patients with solid tumors (generalized malignancy). They were given either an omega–3 oil or a placebo.

The authors found that omega–3 PUFAs had a significant immunomodulating effect and seemed to prolong the survival of malnourished patients with generalized malignancy.

And what of the portion of immune response which we don't want in excess—allergic response and inflammation?

Multiple Sclerosis and Other Diseases of Inflammation

Gently turning the pages of a now-yellowing 1963 copy of *Neurology*, a 1966 article by R.H.S. Thompson, a 1973 article by Tichy and Vyamazal, and a 1983 study by I.S. Neu, one is struck by an important question: What was the common thread here? What had these researchers all hit upon?

People with multiple sclerosis (MS) are low in essential polyunsaturated fatty acids.

If this is the case with people with MS in the general population, then how can DHA help? Well, we must first recognize that MS is an inflammatory disease, a disease which leads to the destruction of patches of fatty myelin sheaths (in brain and/or spinal cord) that enclose portions (axons) of central nervous system (CNS) nerve fibers.

It's possible that the essential fats, such as DHA, can "re-myelinate" some of those nerve fibers or can protect intact myelin from the ravages of the virus, or viruses, which cause MS.

The research

In a 1989 study, University of Minnesota researcher Ralph T. Holman and colleagues examined the fatty acid levels of 14 patients with MS. The results showed a faulty fat-breakdown system, resulting in a low level of omega–6 and omega–3 fatty acids, and a high level of saturated fats.

The authors' observations led them to this hopeful conclusion: "polyunsaturated fatty acid (PUFA) deficiency in MS may be correctable by selective supplementation with PUFA [. . .]. Whatever the cause of MS, accompanying PUFA deficiencies may respond beneficially to nutritional supplementation" with, I must add, omega–6 and omega–3 fats.

In 1990, the English neurologist S. Nightingale and colleagues took up the challenge in their attempt to further clarify the relationship between MS and deficient levels of omega–6 and omega–3 fats. In their research, they studied the red blood cell membranes of 30 patients with mild inactive multiple sclerosis and 30 "healthy" control patients.

At the start of the study, *there was no detectable DHA in any of their MS patients!* Observations such as this led the authors to wonder: "Could treatment with omega–3 fatty acids influence the course of MS?" For their part, English researcher D. Bates and colleagues found the omega–3s to be beneficial in cases of acute, relapsing MS, more so than the omega–6s.

In the Bates's study, which was conducted over a five-year period, 312 people with acute, unremitting MS received either omega–3 fats or a placebo. After 2 years of treatment, these researchers could say, with some context for accuracy, that "there was a trend in favor of the group treated with omega–3 fatty acids."

Other inflammatory conditions: rheumatoid arthritis and asthma

As we discovered in Chapter 1, research over the past 25 years has identified eicosanoids formed from the omega–6 fatty acid arachidonic acid as being on the "Most Unwanted" list of causes of inflammatory rheumatic disease, according to O. Adam in a review article which appeared in the *European Journal of Clinical Nutrition*, in 1995.

What are the root causes? Research has speculated that a virus or bacterium may trigger the activation of certain immune cells, such as B–lymphocytes and T–lymphocytes. This, in turn, may lead to the formation of those inflammatory eicosanoids and cytokines. Studies have also shown that the higher the level of eicosanoids (like prostaglandin E2), the higher the severity of inflammation.

Polyunsaturated fats and inflammatory disease

"PUFAs are the most important nutrients involved in inflammatory distress," Adam pointed out in his 1995 article. In this article, he reviewed current research on the anti-inflammatory diet in rheumatic diseases, and he also described how inflammatory eicosanoids were affected by PUFAs taken from digested foods. As Adam notes, the level of inflammatory eicosanoids (emphasis mine): *depends on* "the amounts, but even more on the *ratio* of the different PUFAs contained in our diet." Further proof that by taking the right ratio of fats we are also opening the door to fighting inflammation and inflammatory conditions!

Like other polyunsaturated fats, DHA's parent alpha-linolenic acid reduces the formation of inflammatory compounds. German researcher, Stefan Endres, M.D., has since concluded that because we now know that interleukin–1 (a cytokine) and tumor necrosis factor (TNF) "contribute" to the progression of inflammatory diseases, consuming EPA/DHA-rich supplements "suppresses the capacity of mononuclear cells to" produce sometimes-proinflammatory interleukin–1 and TNF.

Omega–3 fats (including DHA) have thus been found to protect us against "different inflammatory disorders, such as septic organ failure, rheumatoid arthritis, and asthma," A. Heller and colleagues pointed out in an April 1998 article in the medical journal, *Drugs*.

In fact, a major 1998 study out of the Human Nutrition Research Center, USDA (by Aldo Ferretti and others), which gave DHA to healthy subjects, demonstrated DHA's ability to reduce the levels of inflammatory thromboxane.

Rheumatoid arthritis

Rheumatoid arthritis affects more than 2.5 million people in the United States alone. Most sufferers are all-too-familiar with the morning stiffness, joint swelling, and pain (often of the hands and wrists).

Although its cause is unknown, inflammation in patients with rheumatoid arthritis follows a cascade of cell-cell interactions within our immune system and, specifically, in joint tissues.

According to a presentation given by Albany Medical College's Joel M. Kremer, M.D., at a meeting of the International Congress of the International Society for the Study of Fatty Acids and Lipids (ISSFAL), in June 1995: "Over the past 13 years, or so, about 15 peer-reviewed journals have documented statistically significant clinical improvements in the symptoms of rheumatoid arthritis derived from dietary supplementation with omega–3 fatty acids.''

Improvements have included the following: fewer tender and swollen joints; decreased duration of morning stiffness; increased grip strength; improved joint activity; and extended "time to fatigue." These improvements appear to be accompanied by decreased production, or expression, of pro-inflammatory immune "mediators," such as leukotriene B4, interleukin–1, and platelet activating factor.

The clinical benefits have been found more in patients consuming higher doses continuously for 18–24 weeks. Some studies have even reported on patients who were able to wean themselves off—or even discontinue—those nasty nonsteroidal anti-inflammatory drugs (NSAIDs) after omega–3 supplementation.

Other supplements found beneficial for rheumatoid arthritis include (but are not limited to the following):

- vitamins A, B–complex, C, E
- beta-carotene
- copper, zinc, and selenium
- papain and bromelain
- extracts from birch tree, St. John's wort, and stinging nettle

Asthma and other allergic conditions and crises

According to Australian medical researchers P.N. Black and S. Sharpe, in a review which appeared in 1997, the past 20 years have witnessed an increase in the incidence (and prevalence) of eczema, ulcerative colitis, psoriasis, septic organ failure, allergic rhinitis, and asthma.

Black and Sharpe see that this has been paralleled by a drop "in the consumption of saturated fat and an increase in the amount of polyunsaturated fat in the diet.''

Chart 10.1
Diet Recommendations in Rheumatic Diseases

- Limit omega–6 intake
- Take DHA
- Avoid animal fat intake, and prefer omega–3-rich plants, like soybeans, flaxseed oil, pumpkin seed oil and hemp oil
- Consume foods rich in antioxidant vitamins C and E
- Avoid alcoholic beverages
- Eat high-calcium, low-phosphorous foods
- Supplement with antioxidant vitamins and the trace mineral selenium

As Black and Sharpe explain it, this increase in the diseases just mentioned "is due to a reduction in the consumption of animal fat and an increase in the use of margarine and vegetable oils containing omega–6" PUFAs.

The authors blame the excess consumption of omega–6 fats for much of industrialized society's panoply of allergic conditions and the attendant overproduction of omega–6 derived inflammatory prostaglandins.

Finally, Black and Sharpe attribute the increased incidence here, at least partly, to "allergic sensitization" caused by continually heightened levels of inflammatory eicosanoids, which are then kept "hopped up" by excess consumption of, you guessed it: omega–6 fats.

Inflammatory bowel disease: ulcerative colitis and Crohn's disease

Ulcerative colitis and Crohn's disease are both marked by elevated levels of prostaglandins (especially prostaglandin E2), leukotriene B4, and platelet activating factor.

In 1995, also at the ISSFAL meeting, William Stenson, M.D., of the Jewish Hospital of St. Louis at Washington University Medical Center, reported his results on 24 patients with active ulcerative colitis, whose treatment with prednisone and sulfasalazine was continued during the study.

In fact, Dr. Stenson gave the omega–3 parent compound of DHA, EPA, to the study group, while giving only vegetable oil to the placebo group.

His findings are more than intriguing: Supplementation with DHA, a parent fat, resulted in a "significant decrease" in leukotriene B–4 levels, clinical improvements, and decreased need for steroids in patients with this form of colitis.

Respiratory diseases: asthma

Another group of diseases, themselves caused by inflammation, affect the respiratory system, including asthma.

According to an April 24, 1998, report from the Centers for Disease Control and Prevention, asthma is "one of the most common chronic diseases in the United States, and it has increased in importance" in the past 20 years. The report found that asthma has been increasing in prevalence and in the number of deaths it causes.

While there were "only" 6,770,000 cases of self-reported asthma, in the United States in 1980, that figure jumped to 13,690,000 from 1993 to 1994.

In response to this near doubling of self-reported cases of asthma, a landmark study was carried out by K. Shane Broughton and associates, and published in the *American Journal of Clinical Nutrition* in 1997. In their study, 19 nonsmoking patients with asthma were treated with high-DHA omega–3 supplements.

When the ratio of omega–3 to omega–6 fats was increased to 1:2, 40 percent of the participants "showed significant respiratory benefit." As a result, Broughton reached this conclusion, which by the way is no surprise to us: "Rather than the absolute amount of omega–3 or omega–6 [fats] ingested, the *ratio* [emphasis mine] of omega–3 to omega–6 PUFAs is the critical factor" in beneficially altering the levels of inflammatory chemicals.

They further concluded that "the incorporation of [DHA-rich omega–3 supplements] could alleviate minor respiratory problems in asthmatics or decrease the degree of respiratory problems among a subset of severe asthmatics." And: "these findings raise the conclusion that dietary supplementation [with omega–3s] may be another viable treatment modality for asthma." Pretty impressive findings.

Skin inflammatory disorders: scaly skin

After ingestion, EPA and DHA are converted by the skin to their respective hydroxy acids: 15–HEPE and 17–HODHE. Their presence seems to serve as the body's own way of suppressing skin inflammation, according to Vincent A. Ziboh, Ph.D., in an address he gave at the ISSFAL congress in 1995.

Dietary consumption of DHA and its parent could serve, Ziboh concluded, to "replenish the skin with these natural and potent substances," and, in this way, offer an "alternative or adjunct modality for alleviating skin inflammatory disorders."

DHA anyone?

References

Adam, O. "Review: Anti-inflammatory diet in rheumatic diseases," *European Journal of Clinical Nutrition* 49:703–717, 1995.

Black, P.N., and Sharpe, S. "Dietary fat and asthma: is there a connection?" *European Respiratory Journal* 10(1):6–12, 1997.

Bates, D., et al. A double-blind controlled trial of omega–3 fatty acids in the treatment of multiple sclerosis," *Journal of Neurology, Neurosurgery and Psychiatry* 52:18–22, 1989.

Calder, P.C. "n–3 polyunsaturated fatty acids and cytokine production in health and disease," *Annals of Nutrition and Metabolism* 41(4):203–234, 1997.

Calviello, G. "Dietary supplementation with eicosapentaenoic acid and docosahexaenoic acid inhibits the growth of Morris hepatocarcinoma 3924A in rats: effects on proliferation and apoptosis," *International Journal of Cancer* 75(5):699–705, 1998.

Endres, Stefan, M.D. "Omega–3 polyunsaturated fatty acids and human cytokine synthesis." Presented at a Meeting of the International Congress of the International Society for the Study of Fatty Acids and Lipids; June 7–10, 1995 [place of meeting not available].

Ferretti, Aldo, et al. "Dietary docosahexaenoic acid reduces the thromboxane/prostacyclin synthetic ratio in humans," *Journal of Nutritional Biochemistry* 9:88–92, 1998.

Gogos, C.A., et al. "Dietary omega–3 polyunsaturated fatty acids plus vitamin E restore immunodeficiency and prolong survival for severely ill patients with generalized malignancy," *Cancer* 82(2):395–402, 1998.

Heller, A., et al. "Lipid mediators in inflammatory disorders," *Drugs* 55(4):487–496, 1998.

Holman, Ralph T., et al. "Deficiencies of polyunsaturated fatty acids and replacement by nonessential fatty acids in plasma lipids in multiple sclerosis," *Proceedings of the National Academy of Sciences of the United States of America* 86:4720–4724, 1989.

Iigo, M., et al. "Inhibitory effects of docosahexaenoic acid on colon carcinoma 26 metastasis to the lung," *British Journal of Cancer* 75(5):650–655, 1997.

Kikuchi, S., et al. "Modulation of eosinophil chemotactic activities to leukotriene B4 by n–3 polyunsaturated fatty acids," *Prostaglandins, Leukotrienes and Essential Fatty Acids* 58(3):243–248, 1998.

Kremer, Joel M., M.D. "Effects of modulation of inflammatory and immune parameters in patients with rheumatic disease receiving dietary supplements of omega–3 and omega–6 fatty acids." Presented at a Meeting of the International Congress of the International Society for the Study of Fatty Acids and Lipids; June 7–10, 1995 [place of meeting not available].

Nightingale, S. "Red blood cell and adipose tissue fatty acids in mild inactive multiple sclerosis," *Acta Neurologica Scandinavica* 82:43–50, 1990.

Noguchi, M., et al. "The role of fatty acids and eicosanoid synthesis inhibitors in breast carcinoma," *Oncology* 52(4):265–271, 1995.

Simonsen, N., et al. "Adipose tissue omega–3 and omega–6 fatty acid content and breast cancer in the EURAMIC study: European Multicenter Study on Antioxidants, Myocardial Infarction, and Breast Cancer," *American Journal of Epidemiology* 147(4):342–352, 1998.

Stenson, William F., M.D. "The role of lipid mediators in intestinal inflammation." Presented at a Meeting of the International Congress of the International Society for the Study of Fatty Acids and Lipids; June 7–10, 1995 [place of meeting not available].

Tsai, W.S., et al. "Inhibitory effects of omega–3 fatty acids on sigmoid colon cancer transformants," *Journal of Gastroenterology* 33(2):206–212, 1998.

Ziboh, Vincent A., Ph.D. "The significance of polyunsaturated fatty acids in cutaneous biology." Presented at a Meeting of the International Congress of the International Society for the Study of Fatty Acids and Lipids; June 7–10, 1995 [place of meeting not available].

CHAPTER 11

....

Cardiovascular health

Our findings must add to the concern that the practice of partially hydrogenating vegetable oils [traditional margarine] to produce solid fats may have reduced the anticipated benefits of substituting these oils for highly saturated fats, and instead contributed to the occurrence of CHD.

Walter C. Willett, M.D., 1993

Cardiovascular health has been a watchword for general health now for years. Recently though, medical researchers have determined that the foods developed to replace foods with supposedly bad fat content are actually worse than what they sought to replace. Traditional stick margarine, which was developed from partially hydrogenated oils to replace butter, is the main culprit here, with other so-called diet foods that use margarine in their preparation following closely behind.

In fact, at the ISSFAL congress mentioned in Chapter 10, Stefan Endres, M.D., pointed out that diets overloaded with vegetable oil omega–6 can influence special immune factors called cytokines—IL–1 and TNF—to *bring on* inflammatory disease, including atherosclerosis.

Atherosclerosis, of course, is that dangerous accumulation of "bad" fats inside large and medium-sized arteries. Further underlining the immunity/cardiovascular connections, atherosclerosis is thought to begin—at specific arterial/vessel sites—after a specific type of white blood cell, the **monocytes,** travel from the circulating blood to the innermost layer of the arterial wall (the intima) and stay put due to contact with special molecules called "adhesion molecules" that grow on cells which line the blood vessels.

Once inside the artery, these monocytes are involved in "courting" low density lipoprotein (LDL or "bad") cholesterol. Buildups of fats then lead to atherosclerotic plaque. Resident macrophages stay inside the arteries where, in conjunction with smooth-muscle cells and endothelial cells, they release free radicals, more cytokines, and growth factors.

In severe atherosclerosis, the space through which blood can flow is restricted (or completely blocked) by the accumulation of these "fat Freddies" just mentioned. In addition, atherosclerosis is also marked by the sticking together of Frisbee-shaped blood platelets forming clumps in a nearly out-of-control manner.

As we know, the accumulation of these fats (plaque) or platelet clumps (clots) can lead to stroke, or, more tragically yet, sudden death (**Figure 11–1**).

Research by Raffaele De Caterina, M.D., Ph.D., presented in 1995, has shown that DHA is the only fatty acid, and the only member of the omega–3 family, that can "substantially" (and beneficially) affect the above goings–on.

How does DHA help?

Well, we now know that fatty acids are able to modify the genetic codes we have inherited. For example, in 1995, Steven D. Clark., Ph.D., suggested that PUFAs can reduce risk factors in heart disease by holding down (suppressing) genes involved in lipid "creation" (fatty acid synthase), and by empowering genes involved in blood cholesterol clearance to "get the fat out" (by increasing the number of LDL receptors).

According to researcher Peter Weber, of the Univer-

DHA Reduces Risk of
Sudden Cardiac Death

- Population-based case-control study n=334
- Seattle, Washington area
- All cases free of prior heart disease
- DHA reduces SCD risk
- DHA reduces arrhythmia

DHA Intake* (mg/day)	Odds Ratio for SCD
0	1.0
20	0.9
65	0.7
120	0.5
300	0.4

* DHA intake as fish

Siscovick et al. (1995) JAMA 274:1363.

Figure 11-1

sity of Munich, Germany, omega–3 fats (especially DHA) do, in part, the following:

- Reduce levels of circulating triglycerides
- Reduce levels of the platelet-clumping protein, fibrinogen
- Reduce high blood pressure
- Reduce insulin resistance (or increase insulin sensitivity)
- Reduce the expression of adhesion molecules
- Relax arterial walls (by reducing constriction)
- Prevent the formation of pro-atherosclerosis and pro-inflammation factors, such as: thromboxane, leukotrienes, platelet activating factor, platelet-derived growth factor, IL–1 and TNF

Again according to Weber, at a 1996 "fats" conference held in Barcelona, Spain, omega–3 fatty acids "exert desirable effects" in preventing atherosclerosis or its further progression.

At a more recent press conference held in March 1997, researchers gathered in New York City to discuss the terrible toll on Americans who die each year of coronary heart disease: some 500,000.

The researchers who attended the press conference made special reference to an additional way DHA helps prevent atherosclerosis: DHA can actually lower the risk for experiencing cardiac arrhythmia, the alteration in the rhythm of the heart that often causes cardiac arrest.

This beneficial effect of DHA ingestion was also discussed, in September 1997, by Alexander Leaf, M.D., and Jing X. Kang, M.D., Ph.D., in an abstract presented at the International Conference on the Return of Omega–3 Fatty Acids Into the Food Supply, entitled, "Omega–3 fatty acids and cardiovascular disease."

For their part, Leaf and Kang suggest that omega–3s (DHA and EPA) reduce the risk for, and incidence of, arrhythmia—and sudden "cardiac" death—by electrically stabilizing every muscle cell in the heart. By separating out into the various phospholipids that the heart muscles' plasma membranes need to function properly, the heart's levels of sodium, calcium, and potassium (the electrolytes) are kept in balance.

The Very Latest Research Bears Out the Earlier Studies

At the June 1998 ISSFAL meeting, held in Lyons, France, William Harris, Ph.D.—director of lipoprotein research at the Mid America Heart Institute in Kansas City, Missouri—announced the following validation of the research: "After a careful analysis of a great many studies, it is very clear that long-chain omega–3 PUFAs [DHA] possess a potent triglyceride-lowering effect."

This is especially significant in light of the fact that contemporary research tells us that heightened triglyceride levels are better indicators, and more powerful risk factors, for heart disease than even LDL-cholesterol levels.

While these newest findings are exciting, let's take a look back at what the research has uncovered in the past 10 years.

Reviewing the Research: 1988–Today

The under-understood women-and-cardiovascular disease crisis

I'd like to reiterate that heart disease is far and away the leading cause of death in women. It really dwarfs all other causes of death. This fact is not well appreciated by the public, and is not well appreciated by women, who tend to perceive cancer, particularly breast cancer, as their greatest health threat.

JoAnn E. Manson, M.D., Harvard University, Schools of Medicine and Public Health, July 24, 1996, Harvard Club, New York

Heart disease and stroke is certainly a story of risks to human health. We are all well aware of the heart risks—and problems—men have. These are well-known, well-studied, well-published, well-reported by the media, and well-understood by the public. But what about heart disease and women?

It is not generally known how often women die of cardiovascular disease. And this remains true despite the fact that heart disease kills one out of three women, stroke kills an additional one out of six women and nearly 50 percent of of all deaths in women are related to cardiovascular disease. In fact, coronary heart disease kills six times as many women as does breast cancer, and stroke kills twice as many women as does breast cancer.

There is an additional tragedy attached to these statistics, and it is this: 63 percent of all women who die suddenly of coronary heart disease reported no previous symptoms of the disease compared to 48 percent in men! Want more? The death rate for black women, aged 35 to 74 years, is approximately *two times* that of white women and *three times* that of women of other races.

Obesity is still a problem

In case any of us were beginning to get the impression that a more balanced approach to fat consumption suggests a stamp-of-approval for obesity in women (or in everyone), research suggests we should forget it.

In a 1990 study, Harvard Medical School researcher

JoAnn E. Manson (quoted earlier) found that, after eliminating smoking as a factor, "even mild-to-moderate [obesity] increased the risk of coronary disease in middle-aged women."

Now, on to the research about cardiovascular health and DHA.

1988

In a 1988 study, by Gregory J. Dehmer, M.D., which appeared in the September 22, 1988, issue of the *New England Journal of Medicine,* 82 patients who underwent coronary angioplasty (repair of a damaged/blocked blood vessel) were assigned to one of two groups: (1) those who received a DHA-containing omega–3 supplement before and after surgery (43 patients) and (2) those who received a standard aspirin/dipyridamole regimen. *The results?* Thirty-six percent of the drug-treated patients developed complications (restenosis), compared to only 16 percent in the DHA/omega–3-supplemented patients—who took the supplement 1 week before the angioplasty and for 6 months after.

1990

In the journal, *Atherosclerosis,* the noted German cardiovascular researcher P. Singer (and colleagues) confirmed the lipid- and blood-pressure-lowering effects of supplementary omega–3 fats in 30 male patients with hyperlipoproteinemia. According to the authors, the "most remarkable finding" was a "substantial" decrease in circulating fats and serum triglycerides.

1996

Alexander Leaf, M.D., and Jing X. Kang, M.D., Ph.D., reviewed and examined the anti-arrhythmia effects of PUFAs, and came to this conclusion: "With some 250,000 individuals in the United States, alone, dying annually within an hour of their heart attacks, [. . .]

PUFAs may provide a significant health benefit" [emphasis mine].

1996

Since it's known that vegetarians are typically deficient in DHA, Bruce J. Holub and Julie Conquer, from Ontario's University of Guelph, gave DHA, or a corn-oil dummy capsule, to 24 healthy vegetarians (12 male and 12 female).

Results? The algae-source-DHA-eaters had their serum phospholipid levels increase by 246 percent and their platelet phospholipid levels increase by 225 percent. The authors concluded that "DHA supplementation markedly enhanced DHA status [. . .] and lowered the total and LDL-cholesterol [levels]."

1996

The 610 patients undergoing coronary artery bypass surgery received either conventional drugs or a concentrated omega–3 fatty acid supplement (although all patients also randomly received aspirin or warfarin). In patients undergoing bypass surgery, Norwegian researchers, Jan Eritsland, M.D., and associates found that "dietary supplementation with omega–3 fatty acids" significantly reduced the incidence of complications, such as vein-graft occlusion. The authors concluded that "patients undergoing coronary bypass surgery should be encouraged to keep a high dietary intake of omega–3 fatty acids."

1996

Of 8,006 original participants in the Honolulu Heart Program—who were born between 1900 and 1919—postmortem biopsies were performed on 242 of 1,515 who passed away during the period from 1965 to 1984. Of these 242, 120 autopsies were on men who did *not* have moderate, or severe, coronary atherosclerosis.

The pupose of the study was to look at the development of heart lesions (myocardial lesions) and two factors: smoking and fish consumption. What the researchers found was that smokers who had had 20 years of smoking under their belt had a 50 percent greater risk of myocardial lesions. They also found that participants who had eaten fish at least twice a week had a 65 percent reduction in risk, this effect most evident in subjects who didn't have hypertension. The artery membrane protecting effects suggested by the authors are attributable, clearly, to omega–3 fatty acids, with DHA being key.

The results do *not* mean that we can smoke to our heart's content and solve everything by taking DHA supplements or by eating fish. They merely show that we can reduce a bit of smoking's pattern of destruction by consuming DHA-rich products. The authors' message is very clear: Consume DHA-rich products (in this case, fish) until you quit smoking, but quit smoking as quickly and conclusively as possible, or risk smoking's deadly bag of tricks, including chronic obstructive pulmonary disease and lung cancer, to name only two.

1997

William S. Harris published a meta-analysis or overview of other studies, in which he examined 68 individual research studies that used DHA-rich fish oil, omega-rich flaxseed oil, or a dummy pill. Earlier studies suggested that the effect of omega–3 fats on triglyceride levels (triglyceride levels being even more important indicators than cholesterol) was equivalent to the effect of seed-oil-based omega–6 oils. Harris found more.

Marine oils stronger than land-based? Interestingly, flaxseed oil, which is, for a land-based plant, very rich in alpha-linolenic acid (the grandfather of DHA), does not really decrease triglyceride levels until very large quantities of flaxseed oil are consumed, Harris explains.

Harris added that "the effects of omega–3 fatty acids are now well-established; what remains is to determine the mechanisms behind these effects and, more importantly, their health consequences."

1997

In this year, an interesting DHA study by G. J. Nelson and others came out of the USDA's Western Human Nutrition Research Center in San Francisco.

In a small group of patients, dietary DHA lowered plasma triglyceride levels without EPA, which showed that pure DHA supplementation lowers triglycerides all by itself, without any additional help. Interestingly, a portion of DHA seems to become "retro-converted," or shortened, back to EPA. Regardless, the authors concluded that "DHA can be a safe, and perhaps beneficial, supplement to human diets."

The authors also suggested that "DHA may be beneficial in altering [. . .] cardiovascular disease risk profiles [. . .] with respect to lipids that are risk factors for cardiovascular disease."

Pretty impressive findings.

1997: Ratio, ratio, ratio!

In further proof of our concept that the *balance* of fats is much more important than total fat intake in both men and women, a landmark study came out in the *New England Journal of Medicine* on November 20, 1997.

In this study, 80,082 women were studied who, in 1980, did not have any sign or history of coronary disease, stroke, cancer, hypercholesterolemia, or diabetes. In 14 years of follow-up, the authors documented 939 cases of nonfatal myocardial infarction or death from coronary heart disease.

The upshot? Total consumption of fat was "not significantly" related with the risk of coronary disease.

Based on the consumption levels of trans fats in reference to coronary incidents, the authors calculated that replacing a portion of trans fats (like margarine and other partially hydrogenated oils) with monounsaturated fats (like olive oil) and polyunsaturated fats (like DHA) *"would decrease risk by 53 percent"!*

Having previously reported on the dangers of trans fats in 1993, these results both extended and confirmed the earlier findings. Finally, this landmark study concluded that: "Replacing [trans fats] with" monounsaturated and polyunsaturated "fats is *more effective in preventing coronary heart disease in women than reducing overall fat intake.*"

This truth was echoed at a March 13, 1997, Washington, D.C., symposium, entitled "Healthy Women 2000—Nutrition and Healthy Lifestyles," which was sponsored by the U.S. Public Health Service's Office on Women's Health. At the symposium, Penn State's Penny Kris-Etherton, Ph.D., R.D., discussed the myths and realities of bad fats, emphasizing that, once again, a balance of fats is what's important.

1998

At the June 1998 meeting of ISSFAL, triglycerides were inescapably identified as the main indicators of—and risk factors of—coronary heart disease. In fact, the University of Maryland's Michael Miller, M.D., presented results from his Baltimore Observational Long-Term Study (COLTS), results which showed "elevated triglycerides were a significant predictor of new coronary disease events." He found that study participants with the highest triglyceride levels were "twice as likely" to have a heart attack, require bypass surgery, or die from heart attack as were those with the lowest levels.

These associations have also been independently validated by other studies, including the much noted Harvard Physicians Health Study, the Tufts Framingham Heart Study, and other large studies.

Omega–3s and DHA to the rescue, again?

You betcha. According to Harris, "after a careful analysis of a great many studies, it is very clear that long-chain omega–3 PUFAs possess a potent triglyceride-lowering effect."

Harris, who, as mentioned earlier, is director of lipoprotein research at the Mid America Heart Institute, at St. Luke's Hospital in Kansas City, Missouri, and who chaired the June 1998 ISSFAL session on triglycerides, analyzed over 70 human studies linking polyunsaturated essential fatty acids and triglycerides.

He found that a modest daily dietary intake of 3.5 to 4 grams of long-chain DHA-rich omega–3 PUFAs resulted in a 25 to 28 percent reduction in triglyceride levels. Patients with severe hyper-triglyceridemia experienced a 25 percent reduction in triglycerides (and a 14 percent increase in HDL, "good," cholesterol) with only two grams of DHA-rich PUFAs per day, which is equivalent to about one to two meals of tuna, salmon, mackerel, and herring.

Since, as we talked about in Chapter 1, high levels of fish consumption are ensnared with a whole slew of potential and actual problems, including increasing your toxic burden—by exposure to the toxins found in fish—supplementation here may be the best answer yet.

So what's the big deal about triglyceride levels, since we can go up to 200 mg/dL with those levels, anyway, right?

Wrong. Triglycerides were treated like "poor stepchildren" among heart-disease risk factors, in fact, not even attracting serious attention *as* risk factors by the mainstream medical establishment until after the 1990s.

Today, of course, we know better and rightly so. Triglyceride levels may offer more sensitive indicators of heart-disease risk factors than cholesterol.

Now while the "normal" range for triglycerides is 50–150 mg/dL, elevations were usually, and all too casually dismissed, even when levels jumped over 200. In fact, unbelievable as it is to us today, medical doctors were traditionally concerned only when triglyceride counts rocketed over 500 or 600—posing a risk of pancreatitis.

The truth is, as evidenced in the COLTS study, heart patients with triglyceride levels *over 100 mg/dL* were twice as likely to have a heart attack or bypass surgery, as were those who had levels under 100.

Postprandial triglycerides and PUFAs

After meals, many Americans have their triglyceride levels shooting through the roof. Not aware of that, the main after-meal (postprandial) concern, again of many Americans, is "which mint do I want?" Unfortunately, triglyceride levels can be dangerously high in people with coronary heart disease compared to people who don't have the disease.

In point of fact, elevated postmeal triglyceride levels are linked to a number of metabolic events that can contribute to the development and progression of atherosclerosis—including increased LDL (or "bad") cholesterol, decreased HDL (or "good") cholesterol, and increased formation of blood clots.

What's a "chylomicron"?

Chylomicrons are microscopic triglyceride-rich lipoproteins that show up in the yellowish body fluid, chyle, and in blood.

Are they a problem? Yes! Recent analyses point to the fact that chylomicrons are one of the direct causes of atherosclerosis by way of the formation of their breakdown products. Apparently, these microfats specifically break down into what are called "chylomicron remnants," factors which can be just as bad as excess levels of LDL. Especially after meals, elevated levels of these chylomicrons may increase the levels of those bad breakdown products, or "remnants."

Omega–3 PUFAs and triglycerides—a macro effect on micro particles

Helen Roche, Ph.D., who hails from St. James Hospital, Dublin, has also contributed her perspective to the triglyceride issue. At the June 1998 ISSFAL meeting, she stated that DHA-rich omega–3 fats reduce excess levels of triglycerides, either by directly decreasing the levels produced or by increasing the amount of triglycerides removed from the bloodstream.

In terms of thrombogenesis (the formation of blood clots) and improved platelet function, DHA also looks very good indeed! In fact, in an earlier Dutch study from February 23, 1990, researchers looked at how DHA affects arterial thrombosis and platelet function in an animal model. The lead researchers, and subsequent authors of the study, C.M. Nieuwenhuys and G. Hornstra, found that DHA does reduce blood clot formation while improving platelet function.

DHA and hypertension

Japanese researchers, M. Hirafuji and colleagues, already noted for their previous experimental studies— studies in which they had shown that DHA holds back the progression of hypertension—continued their work.

In their newer study, in which they treated cultured smooth-muscle cells with DHA for 2 days, they also found impressive results. Their DHA treatment "significantly suppressed" the increase in calcium concentration brought on by angiotensin.

As the authors suggest, these results show that DHA specifically holds back the movement of calcium into cardiac smooth-muscle cells—one of the ways in which DHA is said to block the progression of hypertension in stroke-prone spontaneously hypertensive animal subjects.

Take-Home Message?

Throw away your cholesterol counter; cardiovascular research has issued a new mandate—eat more fat—DHA, that is!

References

Burchfiel, Cecil M., Ph.D., et al. "Predictors of myocardial lesions in men with minimal coronary atherosclerosis at autopsy—the Honolulu Heart Program," *Annals of Epidemiology* 6:137–146, 1996.

Clark., Steven D., M.D., Ph.D. "The role of fatty acids in gene expression." Presented at a Meeting of the International Congress of the International Society for the Study of Fatty Acids and Lipids; June 7–10, 1995 [place of meeting not available].

Conquer, Julie, and Holub, Bruce J. "Supplementation with an algae source of docosahexaenoic acid increases omega–3 fatty acid status and alters selected risk factors for heart disease in vegetarian subjects," *Journal of Nutrition* 126:3032–3039, 1996.

Dehmer, Gregory J., M.D., et al. "Reduction in the rate of early restenosis after coronary angioplasty by a diet supplemented with omega–3 fatty acids," *New England Journal of Medicine* 319:733–740, 1988.

De Caterina, Raffaele, Ph.D. "Fatty acids and the control of the early phase of atherogenesis." Presented at a Meeting of the International Congress of the International Society for the Study of Fatty Acids and Lipids; June 7–10, 1995 [place of meeting not available].

Eritsland, Jan, M.D. "Effect of dietary supplementation with omega–3 fatty acids on coronary artery bypass graft patency," *American Journal of Cardiology* 77:31–36, 1996.

Harris, William S., Ph.D. "Omega–3 fatty acids and human lipoprotein metabolism: an update." Presented at a Meeting of the International Society for the Study of Fatty Acids and Lipids; June 1–5, 1998; Lyons, France.

Harris, William S., Ph.D. "Omega–3 fatty acids and serum lipoproteins: human studies," *American Journal of Clinical Nutrition* 65 (suppl):1545S–1654S, 1997.

Hirafuji, M., et al. "Effect of docosahexaenoic acid on smooth-muscle cell functions," *Life Science* 62(17–18):1689–1693, 1998.

Kang, Jing X., M.D., Ph.D., and Leaf, Alexander, M.D. "Antiarrhythmic effects of polyunsaturated fatty acids: recent studies," *Circulation* 94:1774–1780, 1996.

Kris-Etherton, Penny, Ph.D., R.D. "Dietary fat and calories: disease prevention and health promotion." Address given at Healthy Women 2000—Nutrition and Healthy Lifestyles; March 13, 1997; Cannon House Office Building, Washington, D.C.

Leaf, Alexander, M.D., and Kang, Jing X., M.D., Ph.D. "Omega–3 fatty acids and cardiovascular disease." Presented at the International Conference of the Return of Omega–3 Fatty Acids Into the Food Supply; September 18–19; Bethesda, Maryland.

Manson, JoAnn E., M.D. Address given at a Press Briefing on Women and Heart Disease. July 24, 1996; Harvard Club, New York City.

Manson, JoAnn E., M.D., et al. "A prospective study of obesity and risk of coronary heart disease in women," *New England Journal of Medicine* 322:882–889, 1990.

Nelson, G. J., et al. "The effect of dietary docosahexaenoic acid on plasma lipoproteins and tissue fatty acid composition in humans," *Lipids* 32:1137–1146, 1997.

Nieuwenhuys, C.M., and Hornstra, G. "The effects of purified eicosapentaenoic and docosahexaenoic acid on arterial thrombosis tendency and platelet function in rats," *Biochim Biophys Acta* 1390:313–322, 1998.

Singer, P. et al. "A possible contribution of decrease in free fatty acids to low serum triglyceride levels after diets supplemented with omega–6 and omega–3 polyunsaturated fatty acids," *Atherosclerosis* 83(2–3): 167–175.

Weber, Peter C. "Omega–3 fatty acids in the prevention of atheroclerosis and acute cardiovascular syndromes." Presented at the "Fats of Life" conference; November 1996; Barcelona, Spain.

Willett, Walter C., M.D., et al. "Intake of *trans* fatty acids and risk of coronary heart disease among women," *Lancet* 341:581–585, 1993.

PART V

▼

Maternal and Infant Nutrition

The United Nations' World Health Organization (W.H.O.) and the United Nations' Food and Agriculture Organization (FAO) both recognize the critical importance of maternal nutrition before conception, in the conception period, and of maternal/infant nutrition during—and following—a program of breast-feeding.

DHA is an absolutely critical component of prenatal nutrition. It's essential for the proper development of the brain and retina (vision), related to such indicators as intelligence and academic performance, and for physical development.

Unfortunately, the United States Food & Drug Administration (FDA) has been on a holding pattern on the whole issue of whether to allow across-the-board inclusion of DHA and arachidonic acid in all infant formula sold to consumers in the United States.

In the meantime, the irrefutable benefits of DHA in prenatal/postnatal development continue to be elaborated, and confirmed, in well-designed clinical and epidemiological studies, some of which we'll take a look at.

CHAPTER 12

....

Maternal and prenatal nutrition

During pregnancy, the acquisition of long-chain polyunsaturated fatty acids for placental and fetal development is required. [. . .] There is firm evidence that maternal nutrition and health in the periconceptional period is of crucial significance. [. . .] Poor maternal nutrition or metabolic status at this early stage represents a significant risk of compromising embryonic development [. . .] in a manner which cannot be compensated [for] later.

FAO/World Health Organization
Expert Committee, 1994

During the late stages of fetal development, and immediately following birth, the human brain grows very rapidly. In fact, the DHA content of the fetal brain increases three to five times during the last trimester of pregancy and triples, again, during the first three months of life.

The growth of both the retina and "visual cortex" also depends on DHA. The retina develops very quickly during the final months of pregnancy, and the first six months of infancy.

The W.H.O. Recognizes the Importance of Maternal and Prenatal Nutrition

The United Nations' World Health Organization (W.H.O.) even recognizes the critical importance of fatty acid balance in pregnant women and their developing babies. In fact, in 1994, a W.H.O. expert committee produced a report entitled *Fats and Oils in Human Nutrition.*

The report confirmed an extraordinary fact: "There is firm evidence that maternal nutrition, and health in the periconceptional period [around the time of conception] is of crucial significance" to the future development of a healthy baby.

"Evidence from animal experiments suggests that pre- and post-natal nutrition have pronounced effects on brain lipid composition and learning," the report added, pointing out that low levels of omega–3 fats negatively affect nerve structure, learning, and visual ability.

The United Nations' paper went on to acknowledge that "recent study findings in human infants indicate the essentiality of omega–3 fatty acids and the need for the inclusion of [DHA] in food for infants."

A range of studies has shown, the report continued, that the mother's nutritional status around the time of conception has greater significance in terms of birth weight, prevention of neural tube defects, and non-genetic congenital disorders than nutritional status in the latter part of pregnancy.

"Poor maternal nutrition, at this early stage," the report then warned, "represents a significant risk of compromising embryonic development, cell commitment, and the rate of [growth] in a manner which cannot be compensated [for] later."

Essential Fatty Acids, Pregnancy, and the Developing Baby

During pregnancy, polyunsaturated essential fats play an important role in giving rise to prostaglandins and in serving as structural elements of cell membranes.

Throughout the time the little babies are growing, the essential fatty acid needs of pregnant women and their developing babies are very great, needs which are often not met even in the most advanced countries.

In pregnancy, arachidonic acid (AA) and docosahexaenoic acid (DHA) are acquired by the baby, to the detriment of the woman, assuming she does not have optimal levels of dietary DHA and other essential fats—which is, in itself, quite a fair assumption to make.

Studies also tell of the loss of maternal DHA and AA that occurs during pregnancy (Figure 12–1), which is not compensated for by today's prevailing dietary habits, which are typified by low levels of omega–3 fats. This loss of maternal PUFAs—to the developing baby—during pregnancy justifies DHA supplementation in women who are trying to conceive and throughout pregnancy. As we will see in Chapter 13, DHA supplementation is also necessary for women as they breastfeed and (along with AA) for babies as they're being weaned off breast milk.

Essentially: a loss of fatty acids during pregnancy

In 1991, Ralph T. Holman and others published a study that appeared in the *Proceedings of the National Academy of Science USA*. What they found should be of interest to everyone, especially pregnant women and, yes, women considering pregnancy. In a group of 19 healthy pregnant women, circulating blood lipid levels were examined at three time-points: (1) 36 weeks, (2) during labor, and (3) 6 weeks following birth.

The results were not encouraging. Among the pregnant women studied, the fatty-acid "profiles" all showed deficiencies, with the lack of omega–3 fats especially "severe," due to high requirements of the developing babies.

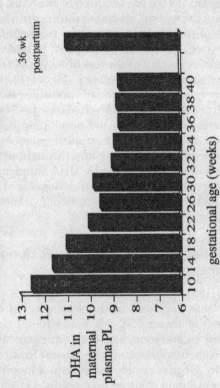

Pregnancy Depletes DHA from Mothers

Figure 12-1

As the authors put it: "During the past 30 years, the control of plasma cholesterol levels by PUFAs, and the consequent decrease in the incidence of circulatory problems have been amply demonstrated, and the food industry has responded by developing oils that are rich in [omega–6] PUFA."

Holman's group then goes on to attribute this poor nutritional status to the dumbing-down of the American diet through cholesterol mania: "Unfortunately, the focus has been on suppressing cholesterol rather than providing balanced essential PUFA [levels]."

The authors concluded that levels of omega–3 fats be increased during pregnancy, when the requirements for omega–3s are highest. As an example, the authors pointed to the development of infants' nervous systems, which are rich in omega–3 fats.

The earlier, the better

"The mental apparatus of the coming generation is developed *in utero*," the authors add. "The time to begin [DHA] supplementation is before conception," when one is planning to conceive.

For babies, the mothers are key

Michael A. Crawford wrote the following in 1991, in an article which appeared in *American Journal of Clinical Nutrition*. It is a statement well worth considering.

The individual responsibility for the development of the brain rests with the mother. Some 70% of the total number of brain cells—to last a life-time—have [already] divided before birth. Indeed, the most active period of brain-cell division is in the first few weeks of embryonic development, almost before a woman knows she is pregnant. At this stage, the nutrition of the embryo is solely dependent on its mother's health, nutrition, and metabolism, because the placenta has not yet formed.

At the completion of prenatal two months, the baby's head makes up almost 50 percent of its body and directs the first movements of the tiny hands and feet. According to Crawford, this is powerful proof of the "overriding priority that human physiology devotes to brain development."

At this point, the placenta takes charge, literally pumping selected nutrients into the growing fetus. It's also at this stage that the developing baby is using up 70 percent of the dietary energy it receives from the mother simply to keep up with its own supercharged growth rate.

Now within the developing baby, the rate of nerve, or synaptic, connections growing between cells is so furious that Crawford estimates a cell may be engaging in "as many as 6,000 to 10,000 connections to other cells" in any one time period. He adds that "the surface area of the membranes constructed to serve these purposes is phenomenal, and makes use of both arachidonic acid (AA) and DHA as basic building blocks."

Crawford's 1989 maternal nutrition and pregnancy-outcome studies

Since there is an association between low birth weight and neurodevelopmental disorders, Crawford and others studied 513 pregnancies in a population in the East End of London, where the incidence of low birth weight is high.

In this study—which appeared in the *Journal of Human Nutrition and Diet*—they tracked 44 nutrients in all of the 513 mothers. Their finding should not surprise us? The authors noted "significantly reduced intakes" of vitamins, minerals, and fatty acids by mothers who gave birth to low-birth-weight babies. Of the 44 nutrients measured in these moms, 43 were below those of the intakes of the mothers who gave birth to babies in the optimum reference range.

The vitamins and minerals most lacking were: thiamin, pyridoxine, riboflavin, folic acid, chloride, and magnesium.

Improve the diet before conception!

Crawford believes that "any intervention to reduce the incidence of low birth weight must be initiated before the mother conceives," especially since "so much brain-cell [development] takes place in the embryo even before the mother knows she is pregnant."

Crawford also went on, in another 1989 study (that appeared in the *Journal of Internal Medicine*), to observe fatty acid levels. Reduced levels of arachidonic acid were associated with low birth weight, head circumference, and placental weight.

Crawford concluded that "maternal nutrition, before conception, is more important than nutrition during the later part of pregnancy, when it is too late to affect the most sensitive period of fetal cell division."

But that doesn't mean that parents should throw up their hands if their baby is born prematurely. Intensive breastfeeding of the baby, supplementing the mother with DHA and a good diet, and weaning the baby (at some point) onto a formula to which DHA has been added are all critical and important.

Do Vegetarian Mothers Need to Supplement with DHA?

In a word, yes. In 1994, Sheela Reddy, et al., from King's College, London, tried to figure out why babies born to vegetarian Hindu mothers of South Asian descent—compared with the general population—were more commonly low in birth weight.

In fact, these researchers found that infant birth weight, head circumference, and length were all lower in this group of women who were vegetarian throughout pregnancy. Although the findings were more suggestive than definitive, these vegetarian mothers did give birth to babies with less DHA in the blood and tissues.

The Dutch studies

Several recent Dutch studies also bear upon our understanding of the relationship between lack of appropriate dietary fats and prenatal development of the fetus. In one study, for example, which appeared in the *British Journal of Nutrition,* Monique D.M. Al and others tried to address what, in 1995, was "hardly any information" about fatty acid status "with respect to the course of maternal EFA status during an uncomplicated pregnancy and its relation" to the newborn's fatty acid levels.

In this study, 110 pregnant women gave repeated blood samples for analysis—from prenatal week 10 all the way through delivery. What did all of the blood samples show? They showed that fatty acid levels "increased significantly during pregnancy," meaning that there was much greater need, on the part of the developing baby, for essential fats, especially omega–3s, such as DHA.

Despite this "maternal mobilization" of DHA, after prenatal 18 weeks, the mother's DHA status declined steadily. Not only did this result in the mother's DHA levels running low throughout pregnancy, it also resulted in a low DHA index in the newborn.

The authors summarized their findings in this way: "It can be concluded that lipid [fatty acid] nutrition of high quality during gestation is [. . .] important, especially with respect to DHA."

Another Dutch study appeared that same year in the *European Journal of Obstetrics and Gynecology and Reproductive Biology*, and featured three of the same authors in the study just mentioned. Were Gerard Hornstra, Monique Al, and Adriana C. Van Houwelingen on to something?

I certainly think so.

In this second study, researchers observed that prenatal development is definitely associated with a high EFA requirement, and, for supply of these essential fats, the developing baby counts on the availability of the mother's essential fats.

Also interesting was the authors' finding that the maternal reduction in DHA levels is not easily made up for after pregnancy. Hornstra and his coauthors suggested that improving the mother's intake of DHA throughout pregnancy will benefit both mother and child.

From all of these studies, then, the conclusion is clear. For women considering pregnancy and pregnant mothers, to ensure the normal development of their babies along with their own health, a balanced diet rich in omega–3 fatty acids is a must. There is no doubt as well that DHA supplementation before and during pregnancy will aid mothers and babies greatly.

References

Al, M.D.M., et al. "Maternal essential fatty acid patterns during normal pregnancy and their relationship to the neonatal essential fatty acid status," *British Journal of Nutrition* 74:55–68, 1995.

Al, M.D.M., et al. "Fat intake of women during normal pregnancy: relationship with maternal and neonatal essential fatty acid status," *J Am Coll Nutr* 15:49-55, 1996.

Crawford, Michael A. "The role of essential fatty acids in neural development: implications for perinatal nutrition," *American Journal of Clinical Nutrition* 57:703S–710S, 1993.

Crawford, MA, et al. "Omega–6 and omega–3 fatty acids during early development," *Journal of Internal Medicine* 225:159–169, 1989.

Doyle W., Crawford M.A., et al. "Maternal nutrient intake and birth weight," *Journal of Human Nutrition and Diet* 2:407–414, 1989.

F.A.O./W.H.O. Expert Committee. *Fats and Oils in Human Nutrition.* Food and Nutrition Paper No. 57. Rome, Italy: F.A.O., 1994.

Holman, Ralph T., et al. "Deficiency of essential fatty acid membrane fluidity during pregnancy and lactation," *Proceedings of the National Academy of Sciences USA* 88:4835–4839, 1991.

Hornstra G., et al. "Essential fatty acids in pregnancy and early human development," *European Journal of Obstetrics and Gynecology and Reproductive Biology* 61:57–62, 1995.

Reddy, Sheela, et al. "The influence of maternal vegetarian diet on essential fatty acid status of the newborn," *Fatty Acids and Lipids: Biological Aspects* 75:102–104, 1994.

CHAPTER 13

....

Infant nutrition

*I will send an angel before you
to the land flowing with milk and honey.*

Exodus 33:2–3

In theory, there is no food better for a baby than mother's milk. Referred to by M. Eric Gershwin as "the natural food of human infants," many of us might believe that it is only a modern-day phenomenon that not all infants are exclusively breastfed.

However, "even in ancient India and Europe, people were taught not to initiate breastfeeding at once," said L.J. Mata in *The Children of Maria Canqué,* "but to give other fluids and other materials, such as honey, substances which were likely to be contaminated; this remains the practice today in many traditional societies."

Infant formulas, in fact, were first used 3,000 years ago, and later became fashionable with European nobility, especially over the past five centuries. Nonetheless, by 1700 A.D., it was observed that feeding children animal milk, rather than mother's milk, brought about a mortality rate of nearly 90 percent. This realization led to the use of wet nurses, who were women brought in to breastfeed the children of nobility. By about 1950, scientists felt confident that they could replace breast milk with low-quality formulas, but they were wrong.

So, as long as every mother nurses, everything's fine? Again, in theory—yes. Without a doubt, if every mother could—and did—nurse her baby, there would be less need for pediatricians in the world.

On the other hand, many mothers, across the board, have poor diets—not only poor women and women in the Third World. They, in turn, pass these dietary deficiencies on to their babies in the form of nutritionally deficient breast milk.

Here are a few scenarios, then:

Scenario 1: Before conception, and throughout pregnancy, the mother has a nutritionally inadequate diet, deficient in DHA. The baby is born early, with small measurements, and is breastfed with nutritionally compromised breast milk. This diet is then followed by a course of formula which has no DHA, whatsoever.

Scenario 2: Before conception, and throughout pregnancy, the mother has a nutritionally inadequate diet, deficient in DHA. The baby is born early, with small measurements, and is immediately placed on zero-DHA formula.

Scenario 3: Before conception, and throughout pregnancy, the mother follows a nutritionally dense, DHA-supplemented diet. The baby is born on schedule, and healthy. The baby is breastfed with breast milk that has a good level of DHA. The mother may choose to supplement breastfeeding with DHA-rich formula, as well. Which scenario would you like to fit into?

Let's take a look at breastfeeding, supplementation with DHA, and traditional formula feeding, and what the research has been uncovering

The Question of Formula Feeding

Eleven percent of the nearly 4 million babies born in the United States in 1994 were premature. A majority of these infants must depend on standard infant formula rather than breastfeeding. Do regular infant formulas provide all the nutrients needed for proper development?

Due to a miscarriage of public health—and to successful lobbying by formula companies who do not want to include DHA in their products—no commercial full-term infant formula in the United States is currently allowed to contain DHA. While formulas do contain the precursor omega–3 alpha-linolenic acid, they don't contain DHA itself. Since infants cannot adequately convert alpha-linolenic acid into DHA, the fact that they contain this parent compound is meaningless. While the neurological benefits of optimal (or even adequate) levels of omega–3 fatty acids (especially DHA) in infancy are most dramatically seen in preterm babies, the benefits are also extremely important for full-term infants.

The Research

A great deal of the groundwork research on fat nutrition in infancy was carried out by Ricardo Uauy-Dagach, M.D., Ph.D, Michael T. Clandinin, Ph.D., and Dennis R. Hoffman, Ph.D., who found that proper visual function and neurological development are dependent on optimal (or even adequate) maternal and infant consumption of DHA.

In 1996, M. Madrikes, et al., also showed that the DHA content of breast milk was directly related to the amount of DHA in the diet. With maternal supplementation of only 200 mg of DHA per day, the levels of DHA in the breast milk were raised by anywhere from 20 percent to 34 percent. The babies of supplemented mothers even wound up with excellent neurodevelopmental results after 1 year of follow-up.

As David J. Kyle, Ph.D., and Linda M. Arterburn,

Ph.D., wrote in 1998 in their contribution to a larger book on omega–3 fatty acids:

> The importance of DHA (and AA) in infant nutrition has recently been made clear with the results of several intervention trials using DHA-supplemented infant formulas. These data have clearly pointed out that formula-fed infants exhibit certain neurological and visual developmental delays compared to breast-fed babies, and when DHA and AA are added to the formulas in the same amounts normally delivered in breast milk, these developmental delays can be minimized or eliminated.

The 1998 milestones in DHA-supportive research

The *Pediatrics* study. There were several ground-breaking studies which came out in 1998, the first of which appeared in the journal, *Pediatrics*. The authors of this study, L. John Horwood, M.Sc., B.A., and David M. Fergusson, Ph.D., reported that in an 18-year study of over 1,000 children, those who were breastfed as infants showed higher cognitive ability in learning and understanding and attained somewhat greater academic achievement than those who had been fed standard infant formula.

The study backed up and extended conclusions of over 20 similar, well-controlled studies over the past two decades which found that breastfed babies have cognitive (learning) advantages over standard-formula-fed babies.

The children who had been breastfed were even 38 percent more likely to complete high school than were the formula-fed kids.

The authors described it this way: "The weight of

evidence clearly favors the view that exposure to breast-feeding is associated with small, but detectable, increases in childhood cognitive ability and educational achievement, with it being likely these increases reflect the effects of long-chain polyunsaturated fatty acid levels and, particularly, DHA levels on early neurodevelopment."

How is this supportive of DHA?

Since the DHA-enriched formulas out there match breast milk levels of DHA, the connection is clear.

The Pediatric Research study

In this study done by E.E. Birch and colleagues, 79 healthy full-term infants received either a standard infant formula (not fortified with DHA or AA) [control group] or the same formula enriched with DHA or DHA and AA for 17 weeks. The visual acuity (vision), growth and fatty-acid profile of these babies were compared—over the first year of life—with those of exclusively breastfed infants.

Results? While the infants fed DHA and AA developed vision on a par with breastfed babies, for those babies fed standard formula visual development was noted as "significantly poorer." To put it in perspective, infants fed standard formula had a visual deficiency of about "one line on an eye chart." In fact, the beneficial "effects of dietary supply of DHA on [visual] acuity were still" evident at 52 weeks [one year later], even though DHA was provided only for the first 17 weeks.

The authors pointed out that these results demonstrate the fact that "the motivation for the assessment of visual function in infant nutrition studies is not" to find massive differences in physical development but, rather, the identification and measurement of "subtle differences," since "even a subtle, or transient, difference in visual function may provide an important clue to the nutritional requirements of the developing central nervous system during critical periods of development." The study concluded that: "Early intake of DHA and AA appears necessary for optimal development of the human brain and eye."

Interestingly enough, the prestigious Nutrition Information Center of New York Hospital-Cornell Medical Center and the Memorial Sloan-Kettering Cancer Center—which is headed by Richard S. Rivlin, M.D., and Barbara S. Levine, Ph.D., R.D.— issued a statement about this study, saying, in part:

> The Nutrition Information Center applauds this research which lends support to our conviction that optimal brain and eye development requires docosahexaenoic acid (DHA). This study supports the conclusion of many other similar well-controlled studies which have been reported in the literature over the last 20 years.

The Lancet study

In this study, 44 term infants were randomly assigned to receive a standard formula or a DHA (long-chain polyunsaturated fatty acid) enriched formula, which they received from birth to age 4 months. At 10 months of age, cognitive (learning) measurements were used to compare both groups.

The results were impressive. The authors found that "an infant's three-step problem solving ability is significantly improved with [DHA and AA-supplemented formula]."

The above are among the many reasons the British Nutrition Foundation, the Joint Expert Committee on Human Nutrition at the U.N. Food and Agriculture Organization (F.A.O.), and the W.H.O. have recommended that all infant formula be enriched with DHA and arachidonic acid (AA).

As of September 1998, 35 countries were distributing DHA and AA-enriched formula for preterm infants, and 6 countries were distributing DHA- and AA-enriched formula (or specialty formula) for term infants. In the United States, this was not the case, at least, not yet.

The United States authorities have been resolutely staying in a holding-pattern on the whole issue, destined, it seems, to repeat the unforgiveable tragedy of folic-acid deficiency and neural-tube defects.

Now the stakes are even broader, on a scale which represents worldwide stunting of brain development, retinal development, and overall neurological development—ranging from subtle developmental differences (representing a few I.Q. points) to serious developmental deficiencies and abnormalities that can and seemingly do occur.

References

Birch, E.E., et al. "Visual acuity and the essentiality of docosahexaenoic acid and arachidonic acid in the diet of term infants," *Pediatric Research* 44(2):201–209, 1998.

Gershwin, M. Eric, et al. *Nutrition and Immunity.* Orlando, Florida: Academic Press, 1985.

Horwood, L. John, M.Sc., and Fergusson, David M., Ph.D. "Breastfeeding and later cognitive and academic outcomes," *Pediatrics* 101(1):1–7, 1998.

Kyle, David, Ph.D., and Arterburn, Linda, Ph.D. "Single Cell Oil Sources of Docosahexaenoic Acid: Clinical Studies." In: A.P. Simopoulos (editor): *World Review of Nutrition and Diabetics, The Return of Omega–3 Fatty Acids Into the Food Supply. I. Land-Based Animal Products and Their Health Effects,* 1998.

Madrikes, M., et al. "Effect of maternal docosahexaenoic acid (DHA) supplementation on breast milk composition," *Europe Journal of Clinical Nutrition* 50:352-357, 1996.

Mata, L.J. *The Children of Maria Canqué. A Prospective Field Study of Health and Growth.* Cambridge, Mass.: The MIT Press, 1978.

Willatts, P., et al. "Effect of long-chain polyunsaturated fatty acids in infant formula on problem solving at 10 months of age," *Lancet* 353:688–691, 1998.

DHA—where do I get it?

DHA, an essential fatty acid necessary for life, is available in a non-fish, micro-algae form. Look for a product called Neuromins® DHA (in softgel form). Because of the importance of this product, several of the leading supplement companies are marketing Neuromins® DHA to retail stores. Listed below are companies—along with their customer service numbers—who can direct you where to obtain this product in your area:

BioDynamax (AMRION):	1-800-926-7525
Natrol®:	1-800-326-1520
Nature's Way:	1-800-962-8873
Solaray (Nutraceutical Corp.):	1-800-683-9640
Solgar:	1-800-645-2246
Source Naturals:	1-800-815-2333
Your Life (Leiner):	1-800-533-8482

Neuromins® DHA is available at healthfood stores everywhere, including the following:

Vitamin Shoppe:	1-800-223-1216
Vitamin World:	1-800-645-1030
Whole Food Markets:	1-800-901-0094
Wild Oats:	1-800-494-WILD

A mail-order source for Neuromins® DHA:

Vitamin Shoppe:	1-800-223-1216

For fish oil DHA products:

Carlson® Laboratories (1-800-323-4141)
PRODUCT NAME: Super DHA™
Available in 500mg softgels

Jarrow Formulas, Inc.™ (1-800-726-0886)
PRODUCT NAME: Max DHA™
Available in 505mg softgels

Feel free to visit your local healthfood store to find the following products, or call these companies to find a store in your area:

Multivitamin and Mineral Formulations:

Carlson® Laboratories (1-800-323-4141)
PRODUCT NAME: Super-1-Daily
Nutrients and excipients derived from sources other than
    animals, fish or fowl. Formulated to contain extra
    Vitamin B-12. Available in tablet form.

Natrol® (1-800-326-1520)
PRODUCT NAME: My Favorite Multiple®
Available in capsules and tablets, also iron-free.

Solgar Vitamin & Herb (1-800-645-2246)
PRODUCT NAME: Omnium Multiple
A complete multiple including Alpha Lipoic Acid and Co-
    Q10. Available in tablet form. Also available in iron-
    free and iodine-free tablets.

Source Naturals® (408-438-1144)
PRODUCT NAME: LifeForce™ Multiple
Metabolic Activator, iron-free, in tablet form.

Children's Multivitamin and Mineral Formulations:

Allergy Research Group (1-800-545-9960)
PRODUCT NAME: Children's Multi-Vi-Min
Developed by Stephen A. Levine, Ph.D. Available in capsule
    form. Also available without copper or iron.

PRODUCT NAME: ProBalance™ for Kids
For children who hate swallowing pills. A great tasting
    combination powdered nutritional supplement.
Blends with any liquid easily for maximum absorption. An
    excellent source of soy.

Carlson® Laboratories (1-800-323-4141)
PRODUCT NAME: Scooter Rabbit
Chewable and tasty tablets containing 13 natural vitamins
and 12 organic minerals. Sucrose-free.

Natrol® (1-800-326-1520)
PRODUCT NAME: A Kid's Companion®
High Potency, Chewable Multi-Vitamin Mineral Formula
Available in wafers.

Source Naturals® (408-438-1144)
PRODUCT NAME: MegaKid™
A delicious chewable multivitamin for children ages 1-10.
Contains a full complement of vitamins and minerals,
and also includes Bioflavanoids, Bee Pollen, Papaya and
Rutin. See bottle for correct dosage according to age.

Balanced B-Complex:

Carlson® Laboratories (1-800-323-4141)
PRODUCT NAME: B-50 Gel
Balanced B-Complex in softgel form.

PRODUCT NAME: Time-B®
Balanced B-Complex in timed release tablets

Source Naturals® (408-438-1144)
PRODUCT NAME: CoEnzymate™ B Complex
Sublingual (dissolves under the tongue and goes directly
into the bloodstream) tablets in peppermint and
orange flavors with Co-Q10.

PRODUCT NAME: B-12
Dibencozide Sublingual CoEnzymated™ B-12.

Natural Source Vitamin E:

Carlson® Laboratories
PRODUCT NAME: E-Gems® All Natural-Source Vitamin E
Available in 30-1200 i.u. softgels.

PRODUCT NAME: E-Sel
Contains 400 i.u. Vitamin E and 100mcg Selenium in softgel
form.

Natrol® (1-800-326-1520)
PRODUCT NAME: Vitamin E 400 I.U.
Available in softgels.

Glossary of selected terms

ADHD attention deficit hyperactivity disorder: one of the most common developmental disorders of childhood (although adults can still suffer with it) which may relate to difficulty in sorting and processing information and sensory data. Diet is a factor too, since ADHD appears to be associated with DHA deficiency, sugar overconsumption, and the toxic burden of artificial food colors and preservatives.

alpha-linolenic acid (18:3w3): the godfather of omega–3 fats, one which yields eicosapentaenoic acid (EPA) and DHA.

ALD: adrenoleukodystrophy (ALD) is a rare, inherited genetic disorder that is marked by breakdown of the fatty myelin sheaths which protect the nerve cells in the brain and by progressive malfunctioning of the adrenal gland.

Alzheimer's disease: low levels of DHA pose a significant risk for the development or progression of this and other forms of senile dementia. Alzheimer's disease is marked by the progressive deterioration of brain tissue, which affects memory, comprehension, speech, movement, and more. It is a devastating and insidious disease which can hit any person, although it usually appears in people over ages 50–65.

arachidonic acid (20:4w6): a key brain fat critical at prenatal and postnatal stages. This fatty acid is often paired up with DHA in DHA-enriched formulas. Excess oil from fish oil can displace ("kick out") arachidonic acid.

atherosclerosis: that dangerous accumulation of "bad" fats inside large and medium-sized arteries, a form of arteriosclerosis also called "hardening of the arteries." It can lead to high blood pressure, stroke, and kidney problems.

cis: refers to the molecular configuration, in this context, of fatty acids—meaning that the hydrogen atoms are all on one side of the double-bond.

DHA (22:6w6): a long-chain, 22–carbon-long polyunsaturated fatty acid with 6 double bonds; the first double bond occurs at the third carbon from the omega end. Found in Arctic/North Atlantic fish; pure sources from ocean-dwelling microalgae are now available.

Depression: in one form is the most prevalent psychological problem in the United States, afflicting about 17 million people every year. It can range from minor "depressive reactions" (temporary states, from two weeks to six months), to "dysthymia" (which may last over two years), to "major depression," a very serious condition that may lead to inability to function and, even, suicide.

Dyslexia: a learning disorder characterized by reduced ability to recognize written words, sometimes marked by the visual "switching" or transposition of letters and words.

eicosanoids: powerful hormone-like compounds which include: interleukins and prostaglandins (derived from "good" and "bad" fats).

fats: called "lipids" by scientists, fats are solid at room temperature; oils are lipids that are liquid at room temperature. Fat is one of six groups of nutrients essential for life. The other five are: protein, carbohydrates, vitamins, minerals, and water.

fatty acid: building blocks which make up fats and oils. Fatty acid molecules have two "ends"—a water-loving end and a fat-loving end. The fatty end is mostly made up of carbon and hydrogen atoms, ending in what is called a methyl (-CH) group. The "acid" end (the water-loving part) is an organic acid called a carboxyl (-COOH) group.

fish oil: although very nutritious, rancidity and contamination remain serious problems with many fish oil products.

Inflammatory bowel disease: any of several debilitating chronic diseases of the gastrointestinal tract marked by inflammation and obstruction of areas of the intestine. Colitis and Crohn's disease are two examples.

JNCL (Batten's disease): juvenile neuronal ceroid lipofuscinosis (JNCL) is marked by rapidly progressive vision failure (optic atrophy) and neurological disturbances.

LCHADD: long-chain 3–hydroxyacyl-CoA dehydrogenase deficiency (LCHADD) is a very rare, inherited metabolic disorder marked by a complete lack of a mitochondrial enzyme which serves as its namesake.

linoleic acid (18:2w6): the godfather of omega–6 fats, one which yields gamma-linolenic acid and arachidonic acid.

long-chain fat: a fatty acid with more than 14 carbons in its chain; most land-vegetable oils we eat are long-chain.

margarine: although some mass-market food processors claim to be "cleaning up their act" by reducing the levels of trans fats in their products, there are so many natural oils to choose from that the choice of margarine, at all, is difficult to justify. The trans fats in margarine make margarine worse than saturated fat ever was.

medium-chain fat: a fatty acid with 6 to 12 carbon atoms. Two examples are: caprylic acid (with 8) and capric acid (with 10).

monounsaturated fats: fatty acids with one rigid carbon link. An example is olive oil.

MS (multiple sclerosis): a disease of the central nervous system, at times slowly developing and erratic in symptomatology. MS causes problems ranging from "minor" physical discomfort to painful and disabling immobility. MS is initially caused by the breakdown of fatty sheaths (myelin) that insulate nerves and provide for the uninterrupted transmission of electrical nerve impulses or signals.

"omega" fats: scientists number the carbon atoms in fatty acids using the "omega" numbering system, starting with omega–1 (at the methyl end) and ending with omega–18 (at the border of the carboxyl end). Omega–3 and omega–6 fats seem to figure most prominently in the human diet.

omega–6 oils: these are the oils most of us associate with land-vegetables and seed oils, including such high-quality oils as: evening primrose, safflower, sunflower, hemp, corn, pumpkin seed, borage, and black currant. On the other hand, highly processed versions of omega–6 oils are what have dominated the U.S. diet for the past several decades, leading to our standing at the brink of "Nutritional Armageddon."

omega–3 oils: these are the oils which are severely lacking in our food supply. Sources include: flax and fish. DHA is one of the omega–3s.

phosphatidylcholine (PC): a key brain neurotransmitter.

PKU (Folling's disease): phenylketonuria is an inherited inability to break down an amino acid. Problems often include: mental retardardation, epileptic seizures, and abnormal brain-wave patterns.

polyunsaturated fats: fatty acids with more than one rigid carbon link. Examples are: DHA, nuts, seed and vegetable oils.

retinitis pigmentosa (RP): a hereditary, degenerative disease of the retina which brings on night blindness, pigmentation changes in the retina, narrowing of the field of vision, and loss of vision.

saturated fats: when carbon links are flexible, the fatty acid is called "saturated." An example is meat fat. We need to curtail the amount of this kind of fat in our diet.

short-chain fats: fat with six or fewer carbon atoms in its chain. An example is butyric acid, a four-carbon fat found in butter.

tardive dyskinesia: movement disorders such as this occur in patients with schizophrenia and manic depression, and are seen in up to 60 percent of people with these disorders who are receiving tranquilizers (neuroleptic drugs).

trans: partial hydrogenation changes naturally occurring cis molecules into what are called *trans* fatty acids, plastic fats whose hydrogen atoms are situated on opposing sides of the fat chain. Some *trans* fats are produced in the rumen of animals by microorganisms, and are found naturally in certain fats, such as beef.

trans fats: found in mass-market varieties of all processed and "refined" foods including: margarine, shortening, prepared mixes, deep-fat fried foods, commercial baked goods (including cakes, bread, and cookies), crackers, canned soups and foods, processed cheese, cereals, candies, mass-market oils, and snack foods. The term "partial hydrogenation" is one of the usual tip-offs that *"trans* fats are served here."

XLRP (or RP): X-linked retinitis pigmentosa.

Zellweger syndrome/pseudo-Zellweger syndrome: a usually fatal genetic disease which ushers in severe neurological symptoms from birth, such as seizures, compromised mental control of voluntary movement, and visual impairment.

ABOUT THE AUTHOR

James Gormley is the editor of *Better Nutrition* magazine, the leading voice in health food store consumer information, a magazine which was founded in 1938 and goes out to nearly 500,000 readers each month across the United States.

His monthly editorials confront critical issues related to health, nutrition, and nutrition politics, while his articles provide insight into the latest breakthroughs in, and understanding of, nutritional approaches to optimal health.

Gormley has garnered GAMMA Awards for Best Editorial Commentary from the Magazine Association of Georgia, both in 1997 and 1998. In fact, in 1998, *Better Nutrition* received the gold General Excellence GAMMA Award and several awards for artistic excellence.

Appearing on major television programs (FOX-TV's "Good Day New York") and nationally syndicated radio ("Shopping Smart With Supermarket Guru, Phil Lempert" [WOR] and "Prescription for Health"), Gormley is regularly interviewed by both nationally syndicated health columnists *(Orange County Register)* and publishing industry sources *(Editor & Writer, Writer's Market, Writer's Digest* magazine).

A voting member of the communications committee of the nation's only health-food-industry trade association, the National Nutritional Foods Association (NNFA), he is also a moderator and guest speaker at key educational symposia and health expos nationwide, including the Hudson Valley Health, Fitness & Nutrition Expo (1997), and key NNFA panels (1997 and 1998).

A former medical/social sciences editor in books, and long-standing member of the prestigious Council of Biology Editors, he has concurrently served as a managing editor of the *American Journal of Surgery* and the *American Journal of Medicine.*

Gormley and family reside in Riverdale, New York.

Index